MICROBES
AND
MINIE BALLS

Microbes
and
Minie Balls

An Annotated Bibliography
of Civil War Medicine

Frank R. Freemon

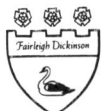

Rutherford • Madison • Teaneck
Fairleigh Dickinson University Press
London and Toronto: Associated University Presses

Associated University Presses
440 Forsgate Drive
Cranbury, NJ 08512

Associated University Presses
25 Sicilian Avenue
London WC1A 2QH, England

Associated University Presses
P.O. Box 338, Port Credit
Mississauga, Ontario,
Canada L5G 4L8

The paper used in this publication meets the requirements
of the American National Standard for Permanence of Paper
for Printed Library Materials Z39.48-1984.

Library of Congress Cataloging-in-Publication Data

Freemon, Frank R., 1938–
    Microbes and minie balls : an annotated bibliography of Civil War
medicine / Frank R. Freemon.
        p.   cm.
    ISBN 0-8386-3484-2 (alk. paper)
    1. United States—History—Civil War, 1861–1865—Medical care—
Bibliography.   2. Medicine, Military—United States—History—19th
century—Bibliography.   I. Title.
    [DNLM: 1. History of Medicine, 19th Cent.—United States—
abstracts.   2. Military Medicine—history—United States—
abstracts.   Z 6672.M2 F855m]
Z1242.F74   1993
[E621]
016.9737'75—dc20   92-52706
                                                                            CIP

PRINTED IN THE UNITED STATES OF AMERICA

CONTENTS

INTRODUCTION

Loud knocking on the door awakened the household. The telegram informed the family that their son has been wounded near Antietam, Maryland. A musket ball went through the neck, but the wound is "thought not mortal." This is the message received by Oliver Wendell Holmes, a leading physician of the era, who immediately began ticking off the anatomical structures of the neck. The telegram was sent by a friend of his son, not by the government. Most people waited until the newspapers published the lists of those killed and those wounded before discovering if their relatives were among the dead or among the maimed.

The impact of the American Civil War cannot be fully grasped without an understanding of its medical aspects. "If its medical aspects are omitted," writes Richard H. Shryock, "the story is not only incomplete but is unrealistic as a total picture." The misery of the battlefield hospital beggars description: the soldier with pieces of bone sticking out of his shattered arm watches the rapid and brutal amputation performed on another soldier; the surgeon wipes the bloody knife on his smock, looks up, and shouts, "Next!" Sam Watkins visits a wounded friend in the hospital; he pulls down the blanket to see that "the lower part of his body was hanging to the upper part by a shred, and all of his entrails were lying on the cot with him, the bile and other excrements exuding from them"— waiting to die. Many grew sick, and some died without ever seeing a wound or even hearing a shot. Debilitating infectious diseases such as chronic diarrhea or malaria afflicted entire armies; scurvy occurred when the armies could not be properly fed. And then the doctors were baffled by a new disease: the soldier awoke feeling fine and ate a good breakfast, but was feverish by noon, delirious by supper and dead by nightfall.

The American Civil War took place during a period of transition between two medical worldviews. The old view emphasized the sick person: he could be restored to health by correcting an imbalance in his system. The new worldview emphasized the entity that caused the illness; a disease was a thing that existed externally to the person, spreading from one individual to another. A disease could be treated by a specific remedy that did not change the response of the individual to other diseases. Quinine was such a specific; it relieved the symptoms of malaria but did not change other forms of fever (according to the old worldview) or other diseases that produced fever (new worldview).

This intellectual transition was a worldwide phenomenon, but American medicine was also undergoing a social change unique to the American condition. In the early days of the Republic, few men held the degree of doctor of medicine. These few had been trained in the great universities of Europe, most notably at Edinburgh. In the early years of the nineteenth century, under the influence of Jacksonian ideology, the old idea of the medical profession as an elite almost disappeared. Many medical schools sprang up throughout the United States, but many were merely a system to transfer fees from student to professor in exchange for a medical degree. By the time of the Civil War, the typical medical practitioner had attended one set of lectures for five or six months, perhaps less, and then, during the following year, he heard these same set of lectures again. He might have been apprenticed to an older practitioner, a remnant of the old medical tradition, but he may have had no apprenticeship at all. Any direct surgical or anatomical training that the medical student obtained were given by some professors for extra money and were not part of the regular lecture series. In short, America had more doctors, but their quality had declined.

In the early nineteenth century, American physicians treated a patient until something immediately visible happened. They bled a patient with a shaking chill until the shaking stopped. They administered a purgative until the patient evacuated his bowels. They gave opium until pain was gone or the patient was asleep. Following the lead of one of the greatest Philadelphia physicians of the turn of the century, Benjamin Rush, they administered their therapies to a degree termed heroic. If the removal of blood from the patient's arm did not stop the chill or lessen the fever, then the doctor withdrew a larger amount. If the patient remained ill after he had been given enough calomel to produce a full evacuation of the bowels, then the doctor gave more calomel.

A reaction to heroic medicine set in, both in the profession and among the public. As described by Lester King, several of the leading physicians of the 1840s and 1850s looked upon Benjamin Rush as the epitome of old-fashioned foolishness. Many diseases were self-limited, these conservative physicians thought, and ran a characteristic course unaffected by any form of therapy. Oliver Wendell Holmes was speaking for this new viewpoint when he claimed that if all the medications in America were thrown into the sea, it would be better for the Americans and worse for the fish.

8

These conservative professional and academic leaders, however, had little effect upon most young doctors trying to practice medicine.

The people of Jacksonian America, like all people, wanted therapy for their ills, both their real illnesses and those that they imagined. Several opposing ideas became popular: homeopathy promised results from minute doses of drugs; botanic practitioners made people feel better with natural products; electrotherapists used galvanism; hydrotherapists applied water. Those who practiced these special forms of medicine were referred to by mainstream physicians as sects or "single idea" men. A group of doctors called "eclectics" tried to use all these therapies.

One heroic idea, the idea of bleeding to restore balance and health, gradually declined and had almost disappeared by the beginning of the Civil War. But the use of heroic doses of medicine, especially the mercury compound calomel, persisted. Medical practitioners thought that they had to do *something* in order to compete with the sects. The medical schools were turning out as many students as would pay their fees, medical licensure laws were lax or nonexistent, and a wide variety of forms of medical therapy competed for public approval.

All this competition made the life of a medical practitioner financially shaky. Some moved to areas of the country thought to be unhealthy hoping that a doctor's services would be in demand. Many people trained in medicine were unable to make a living and gave up the profession. Many doctors only hoped for some sort of regular income. Some became leaders in other fields: a dentist developed the Maynard rifle, and a southern physician used his botanic knowledge to produce writing paper from the okra plant.

In general, southern doctors had a financial advantage when setting up a medical practice. A doctor would agree to treat a plantation family and its slaves in exchange for an annual salary. "Our laboring class is different from yours of the North," wrote Dr. Richard Arnold of Savannah to a colleague in Philadelphia. "The interest, if no other motive, causes the master to obtain medical aid for his slave, and instead of looking to the laborer for his renumeration, the physician looks to the employer. This is the true reason why physicians get into practice more readily at the South than at the North, and that here he stands some chance of making his bread while he has teeth to chew it."

Many doctors in the years before the Civil War sought to practice their profession in the United States Army or in the United States Navy. This career produced a regular income and an opportunity for professional advancement. To enter the medical department of either of the two services, a doctor had to appear before an examining board. The board met once or twice per year, examined all the candidates with oral and sometimes written questions, and ranked them. Only the top few were accepted. A medical career in the army involved many years at the rank of assistant surgeon. Eventually, the assistant surgeon could undergo examination to become a surgeon; this rank was often called major surgeon because it was equivalent in pay to a major of cavalry. The navy had so few places for surgeons that a third rank existed, passed assistant surgeon. This was an assistant surgeon who had passed the test for surgeon, but continued to work at the lower rank while he waited for someone holding the rank of surgeon to die or to retire so that he could replace him.

At the beginning of 1861, the United States Army had just over 100 doctors. Almost thirty resigned when their home states formed a new nation, the Confederate States of America. As the huge armies that would rock North America began to form, many new doctors put on the blue or the gray uniform. Although these doctors bore the official rank of surgeon or assistant surgeon, many had no surgical experience. A large number, perhaps a majority, had never performed any surgery more complicated than lancing a boil. Some had never even seen a surgical operation.

In 1862, the Medical Department of the Union Army went through a vigorous reorganization under its new head, Surgeon General William A. Hammond. Hammond appointed several medical inspectors, equal in rank to a lieutenant colonel, who toured the growing hospital system. Medical examining boards evaluated the new physicians of the volunteer army; many were rejected. Hammond started the Army Medical Museum and the accumulation of reports that would eventually make up the *Medical and Surgical History of the War of the Rebellion*. Hammond appointed his friend, Jonathan Letterman, to the post of Medical Director of the Army of the Potomac.

The Letterman system began in the Army of the Potomac and spread by 1864 to all Union armies. This system introduced standardization: each regiment had an identical medical wagon; each doctor carried an identical medical kit. Medical supplies were stored in excess at many locations in order that they would not be deficient at the key point; "lost supplies can be replaced, but lives lost are gone forever." The Letterman system involved the consolidation of small hospitals to serve each regiment into larger brigade or division field hospitals. The control of ambulances was shifted from the Quartermaster to the Medical Department.

The Confederate Medical Service had even greater problems. From the nidus of a few officers with experience in the old United States Army, the Confederacy built a massive medical organization. The doctors of the Confederacy had a similar educational background to the Union doctors; in fact, a large number had attended medical school in Philadelphia. The Surgeon General of the Confederate States Army was Samuel P. Moore, ranking surgeon from the old army. He screened out inadequate doctors by medical examining boards. He organized the construction of a huge system of general hospitals. The major medical problem of the Confederacy was lack of supplies, particularly of quinine to treat malaria.

Doctors North and South faced the same twin scourges: microbes and minie balls. The minie ball was a cone-shaped bullet that expanded when fired. The expansion forced the ball's edges into the grooves of the rifled barrel; the ball came spinning out of the barrel with greater velocity than the previous musket ball. This gave the weapon greater range, accuracy, and penetrating power. The greater range and accuracy changed tactics: the frontal charge became a massacre. The greater penetrating power affected the doctor who tried to patch up the wounded. Bones splintered, with their jagged ends ripping through flesh. "The minie ball striking a bone does not permit much debate about amputation," concluded Dr. Theodore Dimon.

More important than the enemy you could see were the strange new enemies that you could not see. By the middle of the nineteenth century, medical knowledge was scratching at the new truth that living things could spread disease. Dr. John Gill was amazed when he looked into the clear, rushing water of the White River in Arkansas, but nevertheless knew that "there is something in it that induces diarrhea." John M. Packard painted materials that he called "disinfectants" onto gangrenous wounds to prevent the spread of gangrene to others.

The new medical worldview produced changes in medical treatment. The more advanced physicians, such as J. J. Woodward, recognized that measles was a self-limited disease, infecting each person once and requiring no special treatment; physicians of the old worldview treated measles patients with heroic therapy that produced slower recovery and, in the worst situations, death. The new medical worldview recognized that diarrhea and dysentery were contracted from an unsanitary water supply; sanitation was more important than any pharmacological therapy. The most advanced medical men (and even people without medical training such as General Benjamin F. Butler) recognized that yellow fever could be prevented by quarantine. Advanced medical opinion before the War knew that vaccination prevented smallpox, fresh vegetables prevented scurvy, and quinine taken every day prevented malaria. These truisms were learned again by many physicians during the course of the War.

The War produced another major change in American medicine. In the early Republic, women did most of the nursing of the sick, but this was done in the woman's own home, ministering to the sick of her own family. Hospitals in the early nineteenth century were for transients who did not have family to take care of them; there were almshouse hospitals for the poor, marine hospitals for sailors who had to be left when their ships sailed, and military hospitals for soldiers. These situations had female matrons as supervisors, cooks, and laundresses, but the changes of dressing or the administration of medications were usually performed by convalescents, generally male, who were called nurses. At the beginning of the Civil War, women north and south volunteered for service in military hospitals. Their work produced a change in opinion of the role of women in medical care. After the War, professional nursing began in America as a woman's field.

Did medical and nursing care during the War make a difference? Were more lives saved by proper medical treatment than lost by medical errors? Did the medical system of each side improve the strength of the competing field armies? Did the North or did the South represent the new worldview? Did the successes of the Medical Department of the Union Army contribute to the victory of Northern arms? Did Southern medical successes prolong the war, or did Southern medical failures contribute to the South's ultimate defeat? Did medical care during the War Between the States make any difference at all?

These questions can only be answered by a careful analysis of the primary and the secondary sources gathered in this annotated bibliography. I have tried to reference every letter and diary by a doctor or nurse who participated in the events of the War, even if they made no medical observations. The bibliography includes the most important contemporary medical publications. I have included reports by individual soldiers and officers who were wounded or were hospitalized in order to sample the viewpoint of those on the receiving end of medical care.

The word "minie" was spelled many ways. There is no doubt that the French officer who helped to develop the new bullet spelled his name Claude Étienne Minié with the emphasis on the last syllable. Contemporaries spelled the bullet as *Minié, minie, minnie,* and even *Minnie,* but always pronounced it like "mini-skirt," with the emphasis on the first syllable. The most common spelling was probably minie.

The name of regiments requires explanation. "Fourth Delaware" means the 4th Delaware Infantry Regiment; "8th Illinois Cavalry" means the 8th Illinois Cavalry Regiment. Regiments of the regular army are identified with a number and the name of the nation, as, for example, 2nd United States. Some states provided regiments to both sides, causing difficulties for contemporaries as well as modern readers. One day, the black soldiers of the Union Army's 1st South Carolina gathered for mail call. None of the names called out were members of the regiment. The mailbags had been correctly identified as the 1st South Carolina, but somehow the Confederate and Union mails had been confused. The 1st South Carolina (Union) delivered mail to the 1st South Carolina (Confederate) under flag of truce. This story is related by the nurse of the 1st South Carolina (Union), Susie King Taylor.

The author would like to hear from anyone who thinks a significant source was missed. Every time I have read this bibliography I have discovered errors. Perhaps a few remain; if you encounter one, I would appreciate a communication. The author has tried to maintain absolute neutrality; neither side in this war was all good or all evil. If you write, please inform me if you think I favor the North or the South.

Works by the same author are subarranged by date of publication.

MICROBES
AND
MINIE BALLS

PRIMARY SOURCES

A

Abbot, Samuel L. "Death of Dr. Wm. B. Gibson." *Boston Medical and Surgical Journal* 67 (1863): 324–25.

The author knew William Borrowe Gibson when he had been a medical student and a house officer at the Massachusetts General Hospital. Gibson was a naval surgeon at the siege of Vicksburg when he first developed malaria. Later, while serving with Admiral Farragutt's flagship, the *Hartford,* at Pensacola, he developed a fever thought to be a recrudescence of malaria. While en route home on medical leave, he became delirious and died. He was buried at the Naval Cemetery, Key West.

Abbot, Samuel L. "Air-space in hospitals." *Boston Medical and Surgical Journal* 67 (1863): 403.

A directive of Surgeon General Hammond, dated 24 November 1862, is reprinted with editorial comment. The directive called for proper ventilation of all hospitals. In rooms ventilated by windows, there must be 1200 cubic feet per patient; in pavilion hospitals with better ventilation, there must be 600. The editor does not doubt the wisdom of this order, but its reality. During a recent inspection of Fortress Monroe, the editor noted that the huge post hospital was already overcrowded when it suddenly received a massive influx of patients suffering from typhoid fever and measles. These had just been off-loaded from the ships, and there was no where else for them to go. "Necessity knows no law," he concludes.

Abernethy, Jesse C. "Manual of Military Surgery for the Army of the Confederate States." *Southern Practitioner* 24 (1902): 674–79.

Abernethy was on the committee that devised the Confederate manual of surgery. In this article, he reviews his own book in the light of forty years of progress. "It is strange that our leading medical men," he says, "should be so totally ignorant of the germ

17

theory." He also states that no one in Richmond knew of hypodermic injections. He is quite proud of his clinical description of pyemia, as true today (1902) as in 1863.

ADVERTISEMENTS IN MEDICAL JOURNALS.

Among the interesting advertisements in contemporary medical journals are the announcements for artificial limbs. In 1864, virtually every medical journal carried an advertisement for artificial legs and arms patented by William Selpho of 516 Broadway, New York. These were "the best substitute for lost limbs the world of science ever invented." Another announcement was from Douglas Bly, M.D., 658 Broadway, New York. He advertised "the Anatomical Ball and Socket-Jointed Leg with lateral motion at the ankle, like the natural one." He also carried the United States Army and Navy Leg "furnished to soldiers by the U.S. Government without charge." After the War, these entrepreneurs placed advertisements in the new southern medical journals. Bly opened offices in New Orleans, Memphis, Augusta, and St. Louis. Limbs were for "soldiers furnished on U.S. Government account" (this means for veterans of the Union army) and for "citizens on private account." Southern state governments later paid for artificial limbs for Confederate veterans from their states.

Alcott, Louisa May. *Hospital Sketches.* Edited by Bessie Z. Jones. Cambridge, MA: Belknap Press, 1960, 91 p.

Alcott was a volunteer nurse in hospitals in Washington from late 1862 through the middle of 1863. She has left an interesting description of her daily activities. After serving breakfast to one ward of wounded men, she made rounds with the doctor, acting as his assistant during the changing of bandages and the examination of wounds. Between lunch and supper, she assisted the sick and wounded in small matters, particularly in writing letters. She also kept valuables and keepsakes under lock and key for the patients.

Alison, Joseph Dill. "I Have Been through My First Battle and Have Had Enough of War to last Me." *Civil War Times Illustrated* 5 (February 1967): 40–46.

Although he was a practicing physician, Alison enlisted as a private in the Alabama Mounted Rifles and was sent to the siege of Fort Pickens, near Pensacola, Florida. "I do not think there were less than a hundred fleas on me anytime." In February 1862, he turned in his musket for a doctor's kit and was sent to a hospital in Corinth, Mississippi. Sick soldiers poured in to his hospital; he tried to make them comfortable, but had no bedding or other hospital furniture and very little medicine. Alison accompanied the Alabama Mounted Rifles at the Battle of Shiloh; he dressed the wounds of Federals and Confederates. "I have been through my first battle," he wrote the next day in his diary, "and have had enough of war to last a lifetime."

Alison, Joseph Dill. "With a Confederate Surgeon at Vicksburg." *American History Illustrated* 3 (July 1968): 31–33.

Alison was a Confederate surgeon trapped in the Vicksburg siege. This article contains his complete diary from 17 May to 4 July 1863. The entry from 10 June is poignant: "The wounded are killed in the hospitals, surgeons wounded while attending to their duties. Two days now since Major Headley was killed in camp twenty feet of where I was dressing a wound. Our hospitals are crowded with wounded. Some poor fellows are compelled to lie in the open air and get attention from any doctor who happens to pass that way."

American Journal of the Medical Sciences. Volumes 45–49, 1861–65.

This monthly medical journal was published in Philadelphia. It was the most scholarly medical journal of the era as well as the oldest scientific periodical in the United States. Each issue reviewed major medical and scientific articles published in Europe as well as original American medical science. This journal published the major scientific work on nerve injuries performed by Mitchell, Keen, and Morehouse as well as Austin Flint's essays on conservative medicine. Many issues contain material of special interest to medicine in Philadelphia. For example, the class that graduated from Jefferson Medical College in March of 1861 came from many states, especially southern ones: a total of forty-seven graduates came from Pennsylvania, twenty-six from Virginia, fourteen from Kentucky, thirteen from North Carolina, nine from Georgia and Ohio, eight from Mississippi, seven from Alabama, Tennessee, and Missouri, and six from Indiana and Texas.

American Medical Association Transactions. Volumes 14–16, 1863–65.

The American Medical Association published a volume each year to summarize its annual meeting. The AMA met in 1860 with representatives from every state of the then United States. Meetings scheduled for 1861 and 1862 were cancelled. The first wartime meeting occurred in Chicago in June of 1863. Only representatives of the Northern states were present, but, in the *Transactions,* the individuals who had attended from the Southern states in 1860 were listed as the official, but temporarily absent, representatives of these same states. The AMA took Lincoln's position that the Southern states were still legally in the Union. At that meeting the AMA officially condemned Surgeon General Hammond's action in removing calomel from the army supply table. The most startling event at the 1863 meeting occurred when A. K. Gardner of New York made a motion that medications and surgical instruments should not be considered contraband of war; the United States should allow their importation into the rebellious states. The AMA voted to indefinitely postpone the resolution. The 1864 meeting was held in New York; Gardner reintroduced his resolution, and the AMA took the same action. The 1865 meeting was in Boston. In May of 1866, the meeting in Baltimore welcomed back physicians from the southern states as though they had never been gone.

American Medical Times. Volumes 2–8, 1861–64.

This weekly was published in New York, and some other journals referred to it as the New York *Medical Times.* In the middle of 1864, the increased cost of paper and publishing forced editor Stephen Smith to raise the cost of annual subscription from $3 to $5. Many subscribers failed to renew, and the journal discontinued publication in September of that year. During its existence, the journal carried a weekly column entitled "Army Medical Intelligence," containing orders and transfers of medical doctors, especially those from New York. Occasional editorials made keen observations on the growth of military medicine; an editorial of 30 April 1864 reviewed improvements in the Medical Department of the Army of the Potomac and congratulated Letterman for "his perseverance in effecting these desired reforms."

Andrews, Edmund. "Hospital gangrene." *Chicago Medical Examiner* 2 (1861): 515–16.

The author thinks that hospital gangrene "falls like a pestilence upon the wounded, carrying off hundreds of men who, in civil surgery, might have recovered with ease." He felt that the disease was spread from one patient to another. "No probes or other instruments which have been used in a case of this disease should ever be used on another patient, until they have been thoroughly cleaned by washing, and then dipped in boiling water." He further claimed that the same sponge should not be used on two different wounds; the best cleansing of a wound was not with a sponge at all but with cotton pledgets which can be discarded after one use. Established cases of gangrene should be treated by the local application of nitric acid.

Andrews, Edmund. *Complete Record of the Surgery of the Battles Fought near Vicksburg, December 27, 28, 29, and 30, 1862*. Chicago: George H. Fergus, 1863, 48 p.

Edmund Andrews, a graduate of the University of Michigan, was Surgeon, 1st Illinois Light Artillery. This pamphlet describes the treatment of the Union wounded from the Battle of Chickasaw Bluffs and includes statistics. Troops under William Tecumseh Sherman assaulted the bluffs just north of Vicksburg from 27 through 29 December 1862. They were repulsed, suffering 208 killed in action and 1,005 wounded. [I was unable to read this work.]

Andrews, Edmund, G. H. Hubbard, and Rufus H. Gilbert. "Report of the Committee on Military Hygiene." *American Medical Association Transactions* 15 (1864): 167–81.

This report concerns contaminated air in military hospitals. Air is contaminated by respiration, perspiration, and effluvia from suppurating wounds and bodily discharges. The authors performed experiments to show that the amount of air respired by one man in twenty-four hours is equal to 350 cubic feet. This air "is unfit for any further use; it is deprived of its oxygen." The authors calculate that a ward full of fifty wounded men needs 1.175 million cubic feet of air in twenty-four hours. Only the modern pavilion hospital has adequate air flow; hospitals in large, existing buildings, such as those in Memphis, allow the accumulation of contaminated air. "It is a natural but fatal error for thoughtless or ignorant medical directors to choose for general hospitals the largest, finest, and deepest blocks within their reach, ignoring the fact that the difficulty of ventilating the interior increases as the square of the diameter."

Andrews, Edmund, and John Maynard Woodworth. *The Primary Surgery of Gen. Sherman's Campaigns*. Chicago: George H. Fergus, 1866, 20 p.

Edmund Andrews resigned his position as Surgeon, 1st Illinois Light Artillery in January 1863 and was replaced by John Maynard Woodworth. Woodworth, an 1862 graduate of Rush Medical College, had been a practicing pharmacist in Warrenville, Illinois. He later became medical director of the Army of the Tennessee. During Sherman's march to the sea, Woodworth performed several operations on wounded soldiers including three amputations of the thigh. All of these patients were carried by wagon and did not delay the advancing army; postoperative mortality was zero. The authors statistically compare Sherman's army with other Union forces. [I was unable to read this pamphlet.]

Arnold, Richard Dennis. *The Letters of Richard D. Arnold, M.D., 1808–1876*. Edited by Richard H. Shryock. Durham, NC: Duke University Press, 1929, 178 p.

Arnold was a civilian doctor in Savannah during the War and was also the mayor of that city. He had strong personal and family connections in the North. In a letter dated 14 April 1864, he noted that Savannah's civilian population experienced an increased incidence and virulence of several diseases, including colitis and dysentery.

Arthurs, Robert. "The Man Who Played Doctor: Letter from a Civilian Who Impersonated a Physician in the Union Army." *Civil War Times Illustrated* 19 (August 1980): 36–38.

In a letter, civilian Robert Arthurs tells how he arrived at the Petersburg front and told everyone that he was a contract surgeon. He was given duties examining the wounded and helping to evacuate them to City Point. He never performed any surgery, but he did, according to his account, give surgical advice.

Ashhurst, John, Jr. *The Principles and Practice of Surgery*. Philadelphia: Henry C. Lea, 1871, 1,011 p.

Ashhurst graduated from the University of Pennsylvania with both an A.M. and an M.D. in 1860. He performed several major operations at the Episcopal Hospital in Philadelphia, where he was an acting assistant or contract surgeon, during the War. This work is a huge tome covering all aspects of surgery, described in very plain English. Although the Civil War is never specifically mentioned, the author obviously possesses a great deal of experience in the surgery of combat injuries.

Atlee, Walter F. "Review of Scrive's *Relation Medico-Chirurgicale de la Campagne d'Orient du 31 Mars, 1854, occupation de Gallipoli au 6 Juillet 1856, evacuation de la Crimee.*" *American Journal of the Medical Sciences* 42 (1861): 463–74.

In his review of Scrive's book on French medical experience in the Crimean War, a leading Philadelphia physician makes several comments on the contemporary American situation. For example, in the Crimea, French nuns make good nurses, but the reviewer believes that in the United States, "there are serious objections to the employment of female nurses for soldiers." Detailed statistics show that French troops suffered heavily from disease. About one in four French soldiers who experienced a gunshot wound died from its complications. Scrive recommends amputation for any serious limb wound; he saw many wounded men die, he states, because the surgeon was too conservative. The American reviewer agrees: "The sum of human misery will be most materially lessened by permitting no ambiguous cases to be submitted to the trial of preserving the limb."

B

Bacon, Cyrus, Jr. "The Daily Register of Dr. Cyrus Bacon, Jr.: Care of the Wounded at the Battle of Gettysburg." Edited by Walter M. Whitehouse and Frank Whitehouse, Jr. *Michigan Academician* 8 (1976): 373–386.

Dr. Bacon was assistant surgeon of the 2nd United States during the Battle of Gettysburg. The published diary runs from 2 July to 3 August. The division hospital was set up in the Weikert House where Bacon was assigned as division surgeon. On 3 July, several Confederate shells careened through the hospital area, killing nearby horses; the hospital was moved two miles to the rear. The surgery was performed outdoors, and the wounded were housed in tents gathered from various sources. Rain fell heavily from the afternoon of 4 July to 7 July, soaking everyone. He remained behind while the rest of the Army of the Potomac pursued Lee. His last patients were transferred to the General Hospital at Gettysburg, just north of the town on 31 July. Bacon suffered diarrhea during the later part of his stay at his division hospital. It is interesting to compare his diary notes with his official report in the *Medical and Surgical History,* Medical Volume, Part 1, appendix, pp. 146–47.

Barnes, Joseph K. "The Annual Report of the Surgeon General." *Medical and Surgical Reporter* 16 (1867): 75–77.

This report for fiscal year 1866 contains many statistics from the War. From 16 July 1862, when Congress first authorized the purchase of artificial limbs until the date of this report, 30 June 1866, the Medical Bureau had purchased 3,981 legs and 2,240 arms. During the war, a total of 1,752,377 fluid ounces of quinine in one of four forms had been administered, as well as 2,136,600 quinine pills. In the past year, the Medical Bureau had examined and classified 210,027 medical discharges based upon a surgeon's certificate of disability. The final figures report that 336 doctors lost their lives. Causes of death were:

killed in action	29
killed by accident	12
died of wounds	10
died in rebel prisons	4
yellow fever	7
cholera	3
other diseases	271

In addition, thirty-five doctors were wounded in action but survived.

Bartholow, Roberts. *A Manual of Instructions for Enlisting and Discharging Soldiers.* Philadelphia: J. B. Lippincott, 1863. Reprint. San Francisco: Norman Publishing, 1991, 276 p.

Bartholow was medical purveyor (purchasing agent) with the Army of the Potomac. This work describes the examination to determine if a soldier was fit for service. The first part is entitled "Real Disqualifications for Military Service" and describes diseases arranged by organ systems. The second part is entitled "Pretended Disqualifications for Military Service" and describes how a soldier or a draftee might feign symptoms of various diseases. The third section is dedicated to examining men who are joining the army and the last part to soldiers leaving the army. A major theme of the final part concerns the Invalid Corps, an organization of soldiers who were too disabled to perform full duties, but who could act as guards or garrison troops. The doctor needs to make two determinations: (1) Can the soldier perform full duty? and (2) If not, can he serve in the Invalid Corps or must he receive a medical discharge? A person with epilepsy, for example, cannot perform field service; if he experiences only one seizure per month he can join the Invalid corps, but more frequent seizures dictate medical discharge. Paralysis of one arm is allowable for Invalid Corps soliders; more widespread paralysis is not.

Bartholow, Roberts. "Synopsis of a Report upon Camp Measles, Based upon an Analysis of One Hundred Cases, Made to the Surgeon-General." *American Medical Times* 8 (1864): 231–32 and 242–44.

This long report contains a detailed description of the symptoms of measles. He divides the clinical syndrome into three stages: a formative stage, which continues for five to fourteen days "after exposure to contagion;" the eruptive stage that produces the spots on the body after three days of general symptoms such as cough and fever; and the desquamative stage, which can involve serious complications such as pneumonia or meningitis. After a lengthy description of these complications, including autopsy results, Bartholow concludes that "contagion . . . is the sole cause of the disease." There is no specific treatment, but he gives a wide range of therapeutic recommendations. "Many cases of measles, if left to themselves, terminate favorably by the unassisted efforts of nature." But at General Hospital Number 1, Nashville, where he is stationed, out of 209 measles patients, 42 died.

Bartlett, Stephen Chaulker. "The Letters of Stephen Chaulker Bartlett aboard U.S.S. *Lenapee,* January to August, 1865." Edited by Paul Murray and Stephen R. Bartlett, Jr. *North Carolina Historical Review* 33 (1956): 66–92.

Bartlett graduated from Yale Medical School and, in December 1864, joined the U.S.S. *Lenapee* as assistant surgeon, United States Navy. His ship, a side wheeler of 974 tons and eight guns, proceeded south, and he experienced heavy seas off Cape Hatteras. He was amazed to see the tips of the guns dip under the water with each roll of the ship. His ship and others ascended the Cape Fear River to bombard Fort Anderson near Wilmington, North Carolina. He was on the deck, ready to care for any wounded; "my instruments are sharpened," he said. Noting shells from the fort whizzing past, he concluded that a medical officer was as likely as any ordinary sailor to suffer loss of life or limb.

Barton, Thomas H. *Autobiography of Dr. Thomas H. Barton, the Self-made Physician of Syracuse, Ohio.* Charleston, WV: Charleston Printing Co., 1890, 340 p.

Thomas H. Barton practiced medicine all his life without an M.D. degree. He learned medicine by apprenticeship to his brother, who also never attended a medical school. During the War, Barton was the hospital steward of the 4th West Virginia. He never took the examination to become a medical officer. The 4th West Virginia was formed from volunteers in southern Ohio and western Virginia. This regiment participated in the defense of its home area in 1861 and also in the siege of Vicksburg. The original surgeon of the regiment, George K. Ackley, was a man in his fifties who began to cough up blood (probably from tuberculosis) and had to resign on 11 March 1863. The assistant surgeon, John R. Philson, suffered a severe blow to the head by a falling limb and was never again mentally normal. He was discharged on 3 October 1864. Barton himself lost a great deal of weight from a long bout with malaria.

Baruch, Simon. "Two Cases of Penetrating Bayonet Wounds of the Chest." *Confederate States Medical and Surgical Journal* 1 (1864): 133–34.

The surgeon of the 3rd South Carolina reports the wounds of Confederate soldiers injured during a Federal bayonet charge on 8 May 1864, at Spottsylvania Court House. Two soldiers of the author's regiment were transfixed by a bayonet through the back while lying on the ground. The author administered stimulants to the wounded because of the "shock to the nervous system, induced by the intense excitement of a hand-to-hand conflict with a drunken and infuriated foe." Both patients survived without any surgery. The author thinks that the fear soldiers possess for "cold steel" would be less if they knew that "bayonet wounds are almost harmless when compared to the ploughed tracks which the terrible minie bores through the tissues."

Baruch, Simon. "A Surgeon's Story of Battle and Capture." *Confederate Veteran* 22 (1914): 545–48.

A Confederate surgeon, the father of Bernard Baruch, relates his experiences at Second Manassas, Antietam, and Gettysburg. The first operation he ever performed was on a Union prisoner from Duryea's Zouaves after Second Manassas (prior to this amputation he had never "even lanced a boil"). He stayed behind with the wounded after Antietam; he was taken as a prisoner to Baltimore, where he stayed at the home of Southern sympathizers and had his photo taken while wearing a new Confederate uniform. At Gettysburg, he set up his division hospital in the Black Horse Tavern and experienced an artillery barrage. He remained at that hospital for six weeks and regularly received supplies from Dr. Winston of the Christian Commission. The Union medical director, Dr. Letterman, placed a Union army driver and wagon under Baruch's command. At his hospital he observed six cases of tetanus, all fatal. He was later kept a prisoner in Baltimore for two weeks and exchanged (along with 102 other Confederate physicians who stayed behind after Gettysburg). Much of this material is reprinted in "Bernard Baruch's Father Recounts His Experiences as a Confederate Surgeon," *Civil War Times Illustrated* 5 (October 1965): 40–47.

Baxter, Jedediah. *Statistics, Medical and Anthropological, of the Provost-Marshal-General's Bureau, Derived from the Examina-*

tion for Military Service in the Armies of the United States during the Late War of the Rebellion, of over a Million Recruits, Drafted Men, Substitutes, and Enrolled Men, 2 vols. Washington, DC: Government Printing Office, 1875, 568 p., 767 p.

This statistical material was compiled by the chief medical officer of the Provost-Marshal-General Bureau. The first part consists of physical measurements of a large number of men, mostly those drafted. Most interesting is the average height; the average New England draftee was almost two inches shorter than the average draftee from some of the midwestern states. The information is given by Congressional district as well as by state, revealing, for example, that the average draftee from Manhattan was over an inch shorter than the average draftee from rural New York State. The second part lists diseases and conditions that caused the draftee to be rejected for military service; these are reported by Congressional district, by occupation, and by ethnic group (by European nation of birth). Utilized with proper caution, analysis of these figures could reveal much about the health and nutrition of the northern United States in the middle years of the nineteenth century.

Beach, John N. "Army Surgeons: Their Character and Duties." *Cincinnati Lancet and Observer* 6 (1863): 339–44.

The author, the surgeon of the 40th Ohio, describes why army physicians have such a bad reputation. "Inefficiency, gross carelessness, heartlessness and dissipation are intimately associated in the mind of the Northern public with the medical officers of the army." Many soldiers have died of disease, but fewer, he claims, than in previous long wars. Civilian visitors to general hospitals find a hundred people in a ward much different from a sick room at home. He even relates the story that describes how "a patient in the last agony called the surgeon to him, raised himself in bed, struck the surgeon with all his force, and with a smile of content upon his face, sank back and died."

Beers, Fannie A. *Memories: A Record of Personal Experience and Adventure during Four Years of War.* Philadelphia: J. B. Lippincott, 1888, 336 p.

Mrs. Beers was the northern-born wife of Augustus P. Beers of New Orleans, who served with the 1st Louisiana. She served as a nurse in Richmond hospitals, but followed her husband when his unit was transferred to the western theater. She provides several riveting descriptions: her first exposure to Buckner Hospital at Gainesville, Alabama ("knots of red tape" lead to "supplies scarce, gangrene, foul odors, scurvy, fever, delirium"); the murder of Dr. Francis Thornton (who bled to death in the arms of his wife); the disorganized evacuation of Ringgold hospitals; and her entry into Atlanta by train during the shelling of the city.

Bidwell, Edwin C. "Diagnosis of the Malarial Diathesis: New Test Symptom." *Boston Medical and Surgical Journal* 68 (1863): 36–37.

The author discusses the diagnosis of malaria. While it is usually easy because of the regular intermission of chills, fever, and sweating, sometimes it is mixed with other diseases and diagnosis is difficult. He recommends close examination of the tongue; the malarious tongue becomes thickened and coated. Diagnosis of malaria is important because the disorder responds so readily to quinine and it is so common. "The subtle malaria of the rebel soil destroys and disables more Northern soldiers than all the wounds received from rebel arms."

Bill, Joseph H. "Notes on Arrow Wounds." *American Journal of the Medical Sciences* 44 (1862): 365–87. Reprinted in *Surgery in America,* edited by A. Scott Earle, pp. 228–40. New York: Praeger, 1983.

The author had extensive experience as an army doctor in the west. The first step in treating an arrow wound is removal. An intimate knowledge of Indians is valuable; different tribes use arrows of different lengths. The surgeon puts his finger down the length of the arrow until he finds its purchase. If it is in a bone, great effort may be required to remove it. Bill developed a long forceps with a loop of wire to slide down the arrow shaft if it was imbedded beyond the reach of his fingers. In his career he saw seventy-six individuals wounded by arrows; twenty-nine of these died.

Billings, John D. *Hardtack and Coffee, the Unwritten Story of Army Life*. Boston: George M. Smith and Co., 1888. Reprint. Edited by Richard Harwell. Chicago: R. R. Donnelley, 1960, 483 p.

An astute artilleryman describes the everyday life of the ordinary soldier of the Army of the Potomac. He includes the medical examination of the recruit: "his soundness or unsoundness was then decided by causing him to jump, bend over, kick, receive sundry thumps in the chest and back, and such other laying-on of hands as was thought necessary." He noted that "in 1861 and '62 men were mainly examined to establish their fitness for service; in 1863 and '64 the tide had changed, and they were then only anxious to prove their unfitness." Billings' chapter entitled "Hospitals and Ambulances" provides a brief overview of Union medical care, including the Letterman system. He describes how a hospital tent was heated in winter and the green markings that identified soldiers assigned to ambulance duty. The author concludes this chapter with several eyewitness reports of the care of wounded, especially after the Battle of Hatcher's Run in February 1865.

Billings, John S. "On Medical Museums, with Special Reference to the Army Medical Museum at Washington." *Boston Medical and Surgical Journal* 119 (1888): 265–73.

This article describes the founding of the Army Medical Museum and its subsequent development. Some visitors asked to see the surgical or postmortem specimen of a specific named individual (generally a relative), but this was not allowed.

Billings, John S. "Medical Reminiscenes of the Civil War." *Transactions of the College of Physicians of Philadelphia* 27 (1905): 115–21. Reprinted in his *Selected Papers of John Shaw Billings,* pp. 270–74. Edited by Frank B. Rogers. Chicago: Medical Library Association, 1965.

In the fall of 1861, Billings appeared before the medical examining board of the regular army. He was asked questions for six days, twice the usual period, because, as he found out later, the board had difficulty ordering the candidates: He finished first. The president of the board, Dr. McLaren, asked him to serve at the Union Hotel Hospital in Georgetown, under his direction. Billings had with him a hypodermic syringe; no other physician had one, and it was in great demand for giving parenteral medication (generally morphine for pain). In the spring of 1862, two unidentified but self-important military doctors appeared and examined his hospital. These turned out to be Drs. Letterman and Hammond. Hammond placed Billings in charge of the Cliffburne Hospital, on a hill behind Georgetown. Billings secured sixty Sisters of Charity to do the nursing at Cliffburne. "We should not think them particularly skilled at the present day" he said in 1905, "but they were very good for that period." Cliffburne had a large number of Confederate wounded, who were brought gifts by Confederate sympathizers in Georgetown and Washington. A congressman noted that Cliffburne contained many soldiers from his home district, New York City. "I would like to do something for them," he told Billings, but then added, "something that the papers will notice, you know."

Billings heard complaints that the life of the hospital doctor was soft compared to the experiences in battle of regimental doctors, so he set up a field hospital at the Battle of Chancellorsville. He found that his hospital was too close to the battle line, however; the walking wounded kept right on walking. The band members carrying wounded also passed the hospital, hoping to get farther to the rear, and did not return to try to pick up additional wounded. Billings had great difficulty moving his hospital because ambulances were not under medical control. Billings was also at Gettysburg, where he set up a hospital in a private home on the side of Little Round Top. When shells landed in the area, he evacuated to the rear with little difficulty because he had ambulances under his direct command. Billings noted that the ambulance corps was well disciplined during the Virginia campaign of 1864 at battles such as Spotsylvania and the Wilderness. Billings concludes that the state of medicine and medical education was so primitive, that "it is a wonder that so many of the medical officers did as well as they did, and that the results were as good as they were."

Billings, John S. "An Evening on a Hospital Boat." *New York City Public Library Bulletin* 69 (1965): 308–13.

Some time in the 1880s, Billings wrote out his reminiscences of a boat evacuation from City Point, Virginia. The recollection was partly fictional, since the author had been with the Surgeon-General's Office in Washington throughout August of 1864, the purported time of the trip. The story involves a Dr. McKee, who had treated a large number of soldiers wounded in the Battle of the Crater. They had been under his care at the large tent hospital at City Point, and he obtained permission to assist the naval surgeon during their trip north. The wounded selected were those "so sick or seriously injured that they were not likely to recover for several months, and yet not so hard hit that there would be danger of their dying on the trip." During the boat trip, one soldier developed delirium tremens. Another felt a cramp in his thumb, although the thumb and the rest of his arm had been amputated and, as he said on the ship, "must be fifty miles from here by now." Dr. McKee concludes that, despite the rigors of evacuation, most of the wounded "will have a great story to tell about the mine explosion and their hospital experience, and the little troubles of the voyage will soon be forgotten."

Billroth, Theodor. "Historical Studies on the Nature and Treatment of Gunshot Wounds from the Fifteenth Century to the Present Time." Translated by C. P. Rhoads and introduced by Samuel P. Harvey. *Yale Journal of Biology and Medicine* 4 (1931): 119–48 and 225–58.

Originally published in German in 1859, this important work summarizes knowledge of gunshot wounds just prior to the American Civil War. Billroth, a leading European surgeon, reviews the history of wound treatment and then gives advances of the early nineteenth century. By midcentury, treatment consisted of removal of dirt and debris, removal of the foreign body that caused the wound (if present), and then placement of a dressing. The surgeon might need to make an incision over the ball at some distance from the entry wound in order to effect the removal. The dressing was left in place three days, or ten days according to Larrey, before being changed. In the early nineteenth century, the practice was to bleed the patient. Trephination was performed to remove a foreign body or pieces of skull. Larrey urged immediate closure of chest wounds. Amputation was performed for fracture, especially when the bone broke through the skin. Amputation was performed at one of two times: (1) primary amputation after the soldier had recovered from the initial shock of the injury but before inflammation had begun, or (2) secondary amputation about three weeks later after the generalized inflammation had subsided and the infected tissue had become demarcated from normal tissue. Billroth concludes that recent books on the Crimean War had added nothing to wound treatment. The use of anesthesia is not mentioned.

Boston Medical and Surgical Journal. Volumes 63–72, 1861–65.

During the War, this was the oldest weekly medical journal in the nation. [Continuing today as the *New England Journal of Medicine,* it still holds that record.] Brief summaries of military medical activities emphasized doctors and regiments from Massachusetts. Editorials concerning the trial and conviction of Surgeon General Hammond are interesting. The first, from the issue of 8 September 1864, considers all the charges in great detail and accepts Hammond's guilt: the length of the trial "makes it the more painfully certain that the evidence fully sustained the charges presented." The editorial speaks of "the corruption of so distinguished an official" and "the enormity of the offense." But in the issue of 1 December, the *Journal* published a complete retraction, going over each of the charges, supplying Hammond's defense, and concluding that he was falsely convicted.

Bowditch, Henry I. "Remarks at the Boston Society for Medical Improvement." *Boston Medical and Surgical Journal* (1862–63): 164–66.

Bowditch accompanied a train of ambulances under flag of truce to the Confederate-held Union hospitals at Centreville after Second

Manassas. He was appalled at the disorganization of the ambulance column and the suffering of the Union wounded.

Bowditch, Henry I. "Abuse of Army Ambulances." *Boston Medical and Surgical Journal* 67 (1862): 204–7.

The author continues his comments about the poorly disciplined ambulance service. He recommends transfer of the ambulances from the Quartermaster to the Medical Department. He quotes the report of Major Mordecai concerning ambulance service during the Crimean War.

Bowditch, Henry I. *A Brief Plea for an Ambulance System for the Army of the United States*. Boston: Tichnor and Fields, 1863, 28 p.

The author relates the experiences of his eldest son, First Lieutenant Nathaniel Bowditch, who was wounded in a cavalry skirmish at Kelly's Ford on the Rappahanock on 17 March 1863, one week after the senior Bowditch had delivered an address in Boston on the need for an organized ambulance system. Bowditch went to Virginia to the camp of the 2st Massachusetts Cavalry. He was told his son had been shot in the abdomen and had lain unattended on the field. His unit moved ahead, leaving the field in the possession of Union forces, but no one had been assigned to help the wounded. Finally, a passerby, thought to have been from a Rhode Island regiment, helped Lieutenant Bowditch onto his horse, which had been waiting faithfully. The officer was unable to sit, however, and was draped across the saddle, despite his abdominal wound. He died two days later. Also in this pamphlet is a letter from Charles H. Stedman, who relates how he and the elder Bowditch were at Willard's Hotel in Washington on 5 September 1862 when Surgeon General Hammond asked for medical volunteers to go to Centreville to help the wounded from Second Manassas. He accompanied a Union physician, Dr. J. W. Hastings by flag of truce to the rebel hospital in order to evacuate the Union wounded who had been well treated by the rebel surgeon, a Dr. Miller. Stedman (father of the artist-physician of the United States Navy) noted that the medicine bottles in the rebel hospital all had Philadelphia labels.

Boyer, Samuel Pellman. *Naval Surgeon: The Diary of Dr. Samuel Pellman Boyer,* 2 vols. Edited by Elinor Barnes and James A. Barnes. Bloomington: Indiana University Press, 1963

Boyer was an assistant surgeon serving aboard the U.S.S. *Fernadina* and the U.S.S. *Mattabesett* with the Atlantic blockading squadrons. He had greater difficulty fighting boredom than any other malady. His diary records visits of other naval surgeons, a frequent experience that called for cigars and sherry. He gives the number of the crew sick each day. His second ship became engaged in a gun duel with a Confederate ram. A single shot from the rebel ship, the *Albemarle,* killed two and wounded six of Boyer's shipmates.

Bragg, Junius Newport. *Letters from a Confederate Surgeon, 1861–1865.* Edited by Mrs. Helen Gaughan. Camden, AK: The Hurley Co., 1960, 276 p.

Bragg was surgeon with the 11th and the 33rd Arkansas. Born in 1838, he graduated from Louisiana Medical College. His letters, edited by his daughter, describe military manuevers with little medical comment.

Briggs, William T. "Epilepsy from Injuries of the Head." *Nashville Journal of Medicine and Surgery* 1 (1866): 32–39.

The author reports four cases of epilepsy after head injury with improvement following trephining. One patient had been wounded while serving in the Confederate army—shot in the head at Resaca, Georgia, in May of 1864. The doctor who examined him immediately after the injury thought the bullet had passed through the scalp; he noted that there were two holes in his hat, indicating an entrance and an exit. But for the next two years, this person had continuous infection (called erysipelas by Dr. Briggs) of the scalp at the site of injury and developed epileptic seizures, progressing to a frequency of at least one per day. Dr. Briggs removed some of the diseased skull while his students at the University of Nashville watched. During the exploratory surgery, he found and removed a minie ball that was embedded in the brain substance. Postoperatively, a horrible facial cellulitis developed from the scalp wound. This subcutaneous abcess formation cleared up in two months, seizures stopped, and the patient is now (1866) apparently normal.

Brinton, Daniel G. "From Chancellorsville to Gettysburg: A Doctor's Diary." Edited by D. G. B. Thompson. *Pennsylvania Magazine of History and Biography* 89 (1965)): 292–315.

Brinton entered the Union army in August of 1862 and was surgeon-in-chief of the 11th Corps of the Army of the Potomac. He was a cousin of another leading surgeon, John H. Brinton. His brief description of the surgery after the Battle of Gettysburg is compelling.

Brinton, John H. *Consolidated Statement of Gunshot Wounds.* Washington, DC: Government Printing Office, 1863, 11 p.

This pamphlet, issued as Surgeon General's Circular No. 9, gives a statistical summary of all gunshot wounds treated in United States Army General Hospitals during the last four months of 1862. The number of cases of each type of injury is given, along with much detailed information. For example, thirty-five trephines were performed; twenty-eight resulted in death. The overall statistics for gunshot wounds of all types treated at general hospitals were:

Total cases of gunshot wounds:	20,930
Soldiers who returned to duty:	5,149
Soldiers furloughed:	856
Soldiers who deserted:	374
Medical discharges:	2,897
Deaths:	1,607
Remaining in the hospital:	9,960

Brinton, John H. "Address: Closing Exercises of the Session 1895–96, Army Medical School." *Journal of the American Medical Association* 26 (1896): 599–605.

In a speech to graduating military doctors, Brinton relates several anecdotes concerning the Army Medical Museum. Many doctors opposed the establishment of the Museum, expecting a ghoulish collection of old bones. In August of 1862, the "Museum" consisted of three dried and varnished specimens on Brinton's desk in the Surgeon General's office. But many new specimens came in, and the Museum required its own building: a former schoolhouse on H Street between 13th and 14th. Brinton thinks that medical opinion shifted; the Museum might provide information that would prove useful to future physicians. "Even dry bones may live." The Museum had several early problems. One rough soldier demanded to be given his severed limb that was on display. Brinton deflected his demands, at least for a time, by pointing out that his enlistment was not yet up; he had signed up for three years, his limb was stationed at the Museum for those three years, and it could not desert its post. All the specimens were preserved in alcohol. The great demand for alcohol was met by the provost marshal, who sent to Brinton all alcoholic beverages that were confiscated in Washington. Most of these were redistilled to make pure alcohol, but some of the choicest selections were used for barter. So when the "Museum Messenger" (Brinton) visited front line units to look for specimens, he was a very welcome guest.

Brinton, John H. *Personal Memoirs of John H. Brinton: Major and Surgeon U.S.V., 1861–1865.* New York: Neale Publishing Co., 1914, 361 p.

Dr. Brinton was a Philadelphia surgeon who became a leading medical officer in the volunteer forces. He spent the first year of the war in the western theater. As the Medical Director of Grant's army, he produced a detailed study of gunshot wounds received by Union forces at the Battle of Belmont, Missouri. He was present at the Battle of Shiloh, housing the wounded in tents that had been abandoned by retreating soldiers. He was opposed to women nurses. Later, he was one of the originators of the Army Medical Museum. He spent the last few months of the War in Nashville, where he met the Dr. Cooper who had testified against Hammond in the latter's court-martial; Cooper admitted to Brinton that he had lied to protect himself.

Brown, Harvey E. *The Medical Department of the United States Army from 1775 to 1873*. Washington, DC: Surgeon General's Office, 1873, 314 p.

The portion of this work that deals with the Civil War era is a detailed analysis of medical legislation. The author reviews each act of the United States Congress that influenced the Medical Department. The act of 22 July 1861 increased the number of regular army medical officers, defined the role of the medical cadet, and provided that female nurses could replace soldiers who were performing nursing duties. The act of 16 April 1862 increased the number of physicians further, made the surgeon general into a brigadier general, and added the position of medical inspector. The author also provides details of each medical examining board that examined medical officers for the regular army or for the position of brigade surgeon (a medical officer of the volunteer army not assigned to a specific regiment), including examiners and number of doctors in the regular (not volunteer) army. This is an extremely important primary source for anyone interested in the administrative aspects of Union army medical care.

Bryan, James "Negro Regiments: Department of the Tennessee." *Boston Medical and Surgical Journal* 69 (1864): 43–44.

In a letter from Vicksburg dated 27 July 1863, the author reports the results of his inspection, by order of the medical director, Army of the Tennessee, of the regimental camps of the negro troops. He concludes that "the experiment of making the negro a military power will be a success." He makes several specific recommendations. Too much food is being issued to black troops; the usual government rations "are too large in quantity and too varied in quality for the simple habits of the negro, who does not ordinarily consume as much as the white man." Contrary to popular opinion, the black is not exempt from the local diseases such as malaria. "He suffers from the same maladies, and ought to be treated with the same remedies." The author treated the black soldiers who were wounded in the Battle of Milliken's Bend. [In the same volume of the journal, on page 142, is an announcement that the army needs physicians for the new black regiments. The pay will be the same, surgeons receiving $163 per month and assistant surgeons $112.83.]

Bucklin, Sophronia E. *In Hospital and Camp: A Woman's Record of Thrilling Incidents among the Wounded in the Late War*. Philadelphia: J. E. Potter, 1869, 380 p.

The Soldier's Aid Society of Auburn, New York, sent Miss Bucklin to Washington as their representative. She went to Miss Dix and asked to be a nurse. Although younger than Dix's required thirty-five years, she was assigned to a series of Washington area hospitals: Judiciary Square Hospital, 13th Street Hospital, Seminary Hospital, and Camp Stoneman. She received 40 cents per day. She went to Gettysburg and was nurse in charge of ward B, 3rd Division Hospital, Camp Letterman. On her first day of work, Sunday, she said that soldiers were brought on litters to the hospital, making a line one-and-a-half miles long. She went down the line and ministered to the soldiers: washing faces, combing out matted hair, bandaging minor wounds, and giving drinks of raspberry vinegar and lemon syrup. The hospital was 500 tents set up in neat rows. She thought that the rebel prisoners were more sickly (of the twenty-two in her ward, thirteen died), but obviously believed in their cause and were fierce fighters. Miss Bucklin observed a fist fight between convalscent rebel and Federal soldiers. Both groups were acting as nurses for other Southern and Northern wounded; they had been sent to the cook house to draw rations and not enough was available for everyone. A fight broke out over who would get the rations, the ward of Northerners or Southerners. On this occasion, the South won and scooped up all the food in the cook house. Miss Bucklin was still at Camp Letterman when President Lincoln came to Gettysburg; she heard his address.

In 1864, Miss Bucklin went to White House Landing on the Pamunkey, just after the Battle of Cold Harbor. She saw row upon row of severely wounded and noted that they generally remained silent—unless they became delirious. A pile of discarded limbs accumulated outside the amputating tent. Many wounded had not received care for many days. She opened a wound in one soldier's side to find it full of crawling worms. A doctor poured chloroform in the wound to kill the worms. Then Miss Bucklin cleaned out the huge orifice, filled it with lint, and bandaged it shut just before the soldier was evacuated by boat; she never saw him again. She later moved by steamer to City Point and served at the Depot Field Hospital of the 1st Division, 2nd Corps, where she remained into 1865. Abraham Lincoln passed through this hospital, shaking hands with the wounded, during his visit to Richmond, just before his death.

Buist, Jonathan R. "Some Items of My Medical and Surgical Experience in the Confederate Army." *Southern Practitioner* 25 (1903): 574–81.

Buist was assistant surgeon, then surgeon, of the 1st Tennessee. He rose to be senior surgeon of Maney's Division during the Atlanta campaign. He states that in the early months of the War, his regiment experienced very few camp diseases, because "a large part of the command enlisted out of city population." When he was with the 12th North Carolina, who enlisted from western North Carolina (and were most noted for their accent, especially "we-uns" and "you-uns"), he found that 800 out of the 1,200 came down with measles. In Corinth after the Battle of Shiloh, "nearly all of us had diarrhea and dysentery and a good many were jaundiced." He notes the best method to treat a regiment suffering from diarrhea: move camp. His unit was heavily engaged at Perryville; out of 400 men in the regiment, 50 were killed and 150 wounded. The wounded were cared for in tents or in scattered private houses. One officer received a bullet in the temples that cut both optic nerves; he "lived sightless for 25 years after." Another officer had a bullet wound in the abdomen and survived; the only such survival seen by Buist during the war. He was in charge of the wounded after the Battle of Franklin: 1,500 Confederate and 300 Union. "If I had my service to go through again," he concludes, "I would amputate fewer limbs."

Bumstead, Freeman Josiah. *The Pathology and Treatment of Veneral Diseases Including the Results of Recent Investigations upon the Subject.* Philadelphia: Blanchard and Lea, 1861, 686 p.

This is the standard work on gonorrhea and syphilis, praised by Surgeon General Hammond. Anyone wanting to know how a Civil War physician thought about or treated veneral disease can consult this work. Bumstead does not consider social remedies such as licensing prostitutes. The work went through many editions; the fifth edition in 1883 had grown to 906 pages.

Burton, Elijah P. *Diary of E. P. Burton, 7th Reg. Ill., 3rd brig. 2nd div., 16 A.C.* Des Moines, IA: Historical Records Survey, 1939, 91 p.

Elijah P. Burton was assistant surgeon with the 7th Illinois. This work is a typescript of his diary, running from 7 March 1864 to 22 June 1865. The diary entries are just two or three lines. During the Atlanta campaign, Burton was assigned to the general hospital in Rome, Georgia. The last five pages of this work present a detailed financial accounting of the officer's mess. This diary contains little of medical interest.

Butler, Benjamin F. "Some Experiences with Yellow Fever and its Prevention." *North American Review* 147 (1888): 525–41.

The general in charge of Union forces in New Orleans was faced with the possibility of a yellow fever epidemic. Previous epidemics had shown that the disease was more severe among newcomers, and many of Butler's troops were from New England. He sought medical advice to prevent an epidemic and received two theories: (1) yellow fever was not native to New Orleans, but only appeared when ships carried diseased sailors or passengers; and (2) yellow fever was created and spread by decaying trash. He vigorously pursued a two-pronged effort at prevention: he appointed a doctor to supervise vessels arriving at the mouth of the Mississippi River and to hold all those carrying any person with yellow fever. He simultaneously undertook a vigorous effort to clean up the city. He was very proud that no serious outbreak of yellow fever occurred during the period of Union occupation.

C

Cabell, John L. "Eighteen Cases of Gunshot Wounds of the Head, Observed at the General Hospital, Charlottesville, Va." *Confederate States Medical and Surgical Journal* 1 (1864): 41–43.

Cabell reports eighteen soldiers who received a skull fracture from a gunshot wound. Only three died. Trephination was performed twice, but many patients had extensive debridement with removal of bone fragments, sometimes from the surface of the brain. Several patients had paralysis, usually transient; one patient had a right hemiplegia associated with great difficulty speaking and reading, "from inability to connect the words into a sentence."

Cade Edward W. *A Texas Surgeon in the C.S.A.* Edited by John Q. Anderson. Tuscaloosa, AL: Confederate Publishing Company, 1957, 123 p.

This book consists of the letters of Dr. Cade, who served with the Confederacy in the Trans-Mississippi Department, to his wife, with explanatory material added by Anderson. Cade was born in Ohio, but moved to Texas in the early 1850s. He graduated from Jefferson Medical College in 1858. Many of his Texas neighbors doubted his loyalty to the Confederacy because of his Northern birth and training; for this reason, in late 1861, he traveled to Richmond to offer his services as a doctor. He passed the army medical examining boards, he says, on 29 December 1861; his grade rated him appointment as a surgeon but no such positions were available. He turned down the rank of assistant surgeon and returned to Texas. In September 1862, he again took a medical examination, this time in Little Rock, Arkansas, and again passed. But this time he was appointed surgeon of Randal's Regiment, 2nd Brigade, Walker's Texas Division. He spent the remainder of the War in the Trans-Mississippi theater and has little to say medically, except concerning his own illness of "mucous diarrhea."

Carrington, William A. "Report of Eruptive Fevers Treated in General Hospitals, Department of Virginia, from October 1, 1862, to January 31st, 1864." *Confederate States Medical and Surgical Journal* 1 (1864): 37–38.

The author presents a great deal of statistical material concerning erysipelas, measles, and smallpox. He describes the terrible smallpox epidemic that began during the retreat from Sharpsburg and spread through Charlottesville and Lynchburg to Richmond. The epidemic was at its peak in January of 1863 when 438 smallpox patients were admitted to military hospitals; 221 deaths were recorded. The author quotes Dr. Albert Snead, who had been in charge of the City Hospital of Richmond for 10 years, but had never seen such a fearful epidemic, regarding both the number of cases and percentage terminating fatally. Carrington states that "extraordinary efforts have been made to protect by vaccinating, with pure and reliable virus." He attributes some degree of protection, however, to good ventilation of hospitals and sleeping quarters, which "seems to have so disluted the poison that it could not reproduce the disease in others."

Casler, John O. *Four Years in the Stonewall Brigade.* Girard, KS: Appeal Publishing Co., 1906. Reprint. Marietta, GA: Continental Book Co., 1951, 365 p.

These are the memoirs of a private with the 33rd Virginia of the Stonewall Brigade. His medical problems cut his service short. In August of 1864, when serving in the Shenandoah Valley under

Jubal Early, Casler had a disabling attack of diarrhea. "That night I was taken desperately sick, and I thought I would surely die. I had them get the doctor and he said I had the cholera morbus. He gave me some relief, but I was very sick the next day. It was the worst attack I ever had in my life. It was occasioned, they said, by lying in the hot sun all day." Casler was able to recuperate in the home of a friend, "but had to report to the hospital every day for medicine, as I had the chronic diarrhea." On 19 September 1864, Sheridan's army shattered the Confederates at the Battle of Winchester, witnessed by the debilitated patient. "Early's Army was completely routed, and there is no use denying the fact." Casler fled on foot in order to escape capture. After he felt better, he reported to the hospital in Harrisonburg. "I was not fit for duty in the field," but "I could do duty in the hospital as Ward Master." Later he was discharged and told to report back to his regiment, the 33rd Virginia. His company had completely dissolved, however, so he wanted assignment to the 11th Virginia Cavalry, where he had friends. "As I was familiar with the hospital office," reports the former Ward Master, "I got some blank discharges and filled one out to suit myself." He reported to the 11th Virginia Cavalry but was soon captured and spent the last few months of the war in Fort McHenry, Baltimore.

Chanal, François Victor Adolphe de. "Good Order and Cleanliness: A French Report on Federal Hospitals." *Civil War Times Illustrated* 6 (October 1967): 40–44.

Chanal was an official French medical observer. In 1864, he inspected the Fairfax Hospital, near Washington, and Chestnut Hill Hospital in Philadelphia. He was impressed by their cleanliness and order. This magazine article reproduces his official report.

Chancellor, Charles W. "A Memoir of the Late Samuel Preston Moore, M.D., Surgeon General of the Confederate States Army." *Southern Practitioner* 25 (1903): 634–43.

Chancellor, surgeon-in-chief of Pickett's Division of the Army of Northern Virginia, had great respect for Surgeon General Moore. The author "can bear testimony to his irreproachable character, his energy, and his untiring devotion to duty." Chancellor listed Moore's accomplishments: (1) The use of pavilion hospitals (copied by the North, according to Chancellor); and (2) The establishment of medical examining boards to examine doctors already in service. If the doctor failed, he could serve as a hospital attendant while studying for a reexamination. After a second failure, he was dismissed. Chancellor took the examination himself. Moore's only failing was that at times he was excessively stern and unbending. After the War, Moore did not talk about his military experiences but preferred to look to the future.

Chase, Julia A. *Mary A. Bickerdyke, "Mother"*. Lawrence, KS: Journal Publishing House, 1896, 145 p.

Mrs. Chase interviewed Mother Bickerdyke in Salina, Kansas, on several occasions in 1895. This book about her childhood, early married life, War activities, and postwar experiences can be considered Mrs. Bickerdyke's reminiscences at the age of eighty. Her maiden name was Mary Ann Ball, and she was descended from Mayflower passengers on one side of the family and from a sister of George Washington's mother on another side. As a young woman, she performed volunteer hospital work in Cincinnati. She married Robert Bickerdyke and moved to Galesburg, Illinois. Her husband died in 1858, leaving her with two young sons. She was so involved in healing activities in Galesburg that a city directory in 1860 listed her as a botanic physician.

Shortly after the War began, Dr. Benjamin Woodward of the 22nd Illinois wrote Galesburg citizens a letter asking for supplies. Mrs. Bickerdyke cried when she heard the letter read in her church. She arranged for friends to take care of her children and set off for Cairo, Illinois, with donated supplies for the Union troops there. She was at the battles of Fort Donelson, Shiloh, Vicksburg, Resaca, and Atlanta. She was later at the Grand Review in Washington, setting up tents at Pennsylvania and I Streets to minister to soldiers who became exhausted on the march. The author thinks this act symbolizes her career: while others were receiving accolades from the crowd for their accomplishments, she continued her work of caring for tired, sick, and wounded soldiers.

Chisolm, John Julian. *A Manual of Military Surgery for the Use of Surgeons in the Confederate Army, with an Appendix of the Rules and Regulations of the Medical Department of the Confederate Army*. Richmond, VA: West and Johnston, 1861, 447 p. 2d edition revised and improved: 1862. 514 p. Reprint. San Francisco: Norman Publishing, 1989, 447.

Chisolm had been an observer at Italian military hospitals during the war of 1859. His medical manual became a standard for the Confederacy at the beginning of the War. It includes a great deal of material on administrative medicine—everything from how to record hospital expenditures to the medical organizations of the English and Prussian armies. A second edition was published in Richmond in 1862 and included several new appendices; appendix number 8, for example, consists of food recipes for troops in camp and in the hospital. The work was also published in Columbia, South Carolina, by Evans and Cogswell, 1861.

Churchill, James O. "Wounded at Fort Donelson: A First Person Account." *Civil War Times Illustrated* 8 (July 1969): 18–26.

Captain Churchill was in charge of Company A of the 11th Illinois during the Union attack at Fort Donelson. He was shot in both thighs by pistol balls. He spent the night on the battlefield, drinking melted snow. Blood dripping slowly from his own wound froze into icicles. He was evacuated the next day and placed upon a boat next to the wounded Colonel John A. Logan; Mrs. Logan nursed both wounded men. He refused amputation and was evacuated to St. Louis where he underwent a long and painful recovery. This is perhaps the best description of how it feels to be wounded, to await initial medical care, to be examined by doctors, to undergo evacuation, and to experience prolonged hospitalization.

Cincinnati Lancet and Observer. Volumes 4–8, 1861–65.

This monthly magazine contained much material on the War, particularly as it affected Ohio and other western states. Cincinnati was an unusual medical town, with a great number of irregular practitioners. The city had three medical schools to train young men in nontraditional healing practices: the Electic Medical Institute, the Physio-Medical Institute, and the Botanic-Physic College. The *Cincinnati Lancet and Observer* was edited by and directed to traditional physicians, such as the graduates of the two regular medical schools in town, the Medical College of Ohio and the Cincinnati College of Medicine and Surgery. Surgeon General Hammond's order restricting calomel and tartar emetic was strongly opposed by the *Lancet and Observer,* since the irregular doctors had for many years shouted the dangers of these medications. With this exception, this journal supported Hammond and the Army Medical Bureau and published a very long and favorable editorial early in 1864.

Clark, Charles M. *History of the 39th Regiment, Illinois Volunteer Veteran Infantry (Yates' Phalanx).* Chicago: Veterans Association of the Regiment, 1889, 554 p.

The surgeon of the 39th Illinois writes the regimental history and includes medical comments. The regiment opposed Stonewall Jackson in the Valley campaign of 1862, spent 1863 in South Carolina, and accompanied Butler in the Bermuda Hundred campaign.

Clark, Henry G. "Inspection of Military Hospitals." *Boston Medical and Surgical Journal* 67 (1863): 443–44.

This report described a civilian inspection by a group of leading doctors of Union army general hospitals. Inspectors included Bowditch, Ellis, Stephen Smith, David Judkins of Cincinnati, Joshua B. Flint of Louisville, Charles Ware, Benjamin Shaw, Morreill Wyman, Edmond Fowler of Alabama, Francis Minot, and Samuel L. Abbot. The hospital surgeons-in-charge welcomed the inspectors with one exception, not specified, who was "promptly rebuked by the Surgeon General." Defects discovered by the inspectors were communicated to Hammond and "received his immediate and effective attention." Clark concludes that problems exist in some general hospitals, but one must remember that "to start and put into working order the ponderous machinery of Hospitals which contain, in the mass, more than 70,000 beds, without any friction, would be a miracle. Let us then, instead of criticizing too sharply, rather admire the energy, the skill, the administrative capacity, shown in extemporizing and systematizing an agency so beneficient and so grand."

Clarke, J. H. "Yellow Fever in New Orleans." *Boston Medical and Surgical Journal* 68 (1864): 303–4.

A naval surgeon at New Orleans reports several cases of yellow fever, with nineteen deaths (estimated mortality of 60 percent). All cases were acquired on board ship prior to arrival at New Orleans. Three fatalities occurred among sailors from the ship *De Soto* who were aboard a captured prize ship.

Cleaveland, Charles H. *Causes and Cure of Diseases of the Feet.* Cincinnati, OH: Bradley and Webb, 1862, 111 p.

Cleaveland was born in 1820 and graduated from Dartmouth Medical College in 1843. He died of disease while serving as a medical officer in Memphis. In this work, Cleaveland notes that the War has stimulated interest in foot problems. Infantry soldiers need healthy feet. According to Rutkow, this paperbound volume is the earliest work in America to deal strictly with problems of the feet.

Clements, Bennett A. "Notes of Surgical Cases." *American Journal of the Medical Sciences* 42 (1861): 37–46.

The author was a career medical officer with the United States Army, writing from Fort Fauntleroy, New Mexico Territory, in February 1861. He reports on six unrelated cases encountered mostly during the military action in Utah. One patient received a bayonet wound of the abdomen and recovered. A woman developed a sore on her lip when bitten, in an embrace, by her husband who, at the time, had secondary syphilitic sores in his mouth. The woman later developed secondary syphilis. Clements quotes two articles from the British medical journal, *Lancet,* that claim that syphilis "can be contracted by transmission from secondary sores."

Clements, Bennett A. *Memoir of Jonathan Letterman.* New York: G. P. Putnam's Sons, 1883, 38 p.

A career United States Army medical officer eulogizes the medical director of the Army of the Potomac. [I was unable to read this pamphlet.]

Coles, Abraham. "On Hospital Gangrene." *Medical Society of New Jersey Transactions* 98 (1864): 45–59.

The author, a civilian physician, reviews the literature concerning hospital gangrene. He concludes that the disease most often occurs in debilitated patients. "It is *often* produced by a direct application of the poisonous matter generated by the disease to a wounded or ulcerated surface; in other words it is inocuable and contagious; but this cause does not *always* produce it, nor is it the *sole* cause, as proved by the fact that the first case must necessarily have had some other origin. It is sometimes communicated from one person to another through the medium of the air, but this would seem to be not of frequent occurrence; that is to say, it is occasionally infectious, but not generally so."

Coles attempts to explain how a drop of this poisonous matter multiplies after transmission. He draws an analogy to fermentation, "a peculiar kind of putrefactive fermentation," but he never mentions the contemporary researches of Pasteur. "That first cell-germ with which the process begins may be so inconceivably minute that a pin's point would cover it a thousand times, and yet from that moment the work is begun it goes steadily on . . . until it takes in the whole surface of the original wound, and stops not there, but prosecutes its ravages far beyond." Coles quotes many military surgeons such as Barron Larrey and even the recent researches on bromine as a topical treatment as reported by Middleton Goldsmith, medical director of the Union army hospitals in Louisville. This article is valuable because it records the ideas of an intelligent civilian doctor about contagion and infection. Coles concludes that "we have a great deal to learn touching this whole subject."

Confederate States Medical and Surgical Journal. Volume 1 (12 monthly numbers) 1864; Volume 2 (2 numbers, January and February) 1865. Reprint of the full series, with an introduction by William D. Sharpe. Metuchen, NJ: Scarecrow Press, 1959, 249 p.

Samuel P. Moore, Surgeon General of the Confederate States Army, was the major force behind this work, although he is not listed as the editor and the journal was the official responsibility of a committee. Each issue, about twenty pages in length, is packed with interesting cases and observations submitted by physicians from all over the Confederacy. The editors summarized a few articles published in European medical journals with emphasis upon tetanus and hysteria.

In the first report in the first issue, Joseph Jones reports a 37-year-old private named Gilstrap, who developed tetanus after being shot in the arm. While defending James Island, South Carolina, Gilstrap was in a house. An enemy minie ball pierced the plank wall of the house, estimated as three inches in thickness, and then ripped through his right arm, proceeding between and damaging, but not dividing, the two bones of the forearm. The injury healed well with standard dressings, but about three weeks later, the man developed spasms of all four limbs and contractions of the muscles of his back, neck, and jaw. Jones made the diagnosis of traumatic tetanus and treated him with a mixture of calomel, castor oil, brandy, quinine, and chloroform. The chloroform was given orally, and the patient's urine, which was thoroughly analyzed, developed the distinct odor of the anesthetic. The patient survived.

Almost the last article in the final printed issue summarizes the court-martial of William A. Hammond, the Surgeon General of the United States Army. The brief statement, printed without editorial comment, states that Hammond was cashiered and forbidden to ever hold federal office because he was found guilty of "official corruption, abuse of power, and a gross breach of the public trust." The March issue had been completed and was ready for the publisher, but was destroyed in the Richmond fire of 2 to 3 April 1865.

Conrad, Daniel B. "Capture and Burning of the Federal Gunboat *Underwriter,* in the Neuse, off New Bern, N.C., in February, 1864." *Southern Historical Society Papers* 19 (1891): 93–100.

Conrad was a physician in the United States Navy who resigned to join the Confederate States Navy. This article describes his experience with a small band of men who, under the command of the famous J. Taylor Wood, boarded a United States Navy vessel at anchor to try to capture her. Conrad participated in the raid and treated the wounded. "I examined a youth who was sitting in the lap of another, and in feeling his head I felt my hand slip down between his ears, and to my horror, discovered that his head had been cleft in two by a boarding sword in the hands of some giant of the forecastle." Conrad was fleet surgeon for Admiral Buchanan during the Battle of Mobile Bay.

Coolidge, Richard H. *Statistical Report on the Sickness and Mortality in the Army of the United States, Compiled from the Records of the Surgeon General's Office; Embracing a Period of Five Years from January, 1855, to January, 1860.* Washington, DC: George W. Bowman, 1860, 515 p.

This statistical study reports on the health of the United States Army just prior to the Civil War. Brief reports concerning health conditions at various posts were written by army doctors such as Joseph Barnes, Jonathan Letterman, Lafayette Guild, Roberts Bartholow and B. J. D. Irwin. Yellow fever occurred at Key West and at Fort Moultrie, South Carolina.

Cumming, Kate. *A Journal of Hospital Life in the Confederate Army of Tennesse, from the Battle of Shiloh to the End of the War.* New Orleans: John P. Morgan, 1866, 199 p. Reprinted as her *Kate: The Journal of a Confederate Nurse.* With an introduction and footnotes by Richard Barksdale Harwell. Baton Rouge: Louisiana State University Press, 1959, 321 p.

The author was a very active nurse with the general hospitals of the Army of Tennessee. She was at Corinth after the Battle of Shiloh, at Chattanooga until it was evacuated by the Confederates, and at the general hospital at Newnan during the Atlanta campaign. She accompanied the Newnan Hospital when it was evacuated to Americus, Georgia.

Craighill, Edward A. *Confederate Surgeon: The Personal Recollections of E. A. Craighill.* Edited by Peter W. Houck. Lynchburg, VA: H. E. Howard, 1989, 106 p.

In 1905, at the age of sixty-five, Dr. Craighill wrote his memories of his Confederate service. Born and raised in the northern portion of the Shenandoah Valley, he graduated from the medical school of the University of Pennsylvania in the class of 1861 at the age of twenty. He enlisted as a private in the local company, which became part of the 2nd Virginia. Dr. Hunter Holmes McGuire, who had known Craighill both as a child and when they were both medical students at Pennsylvania, arranged for the new medical graduate to become a hospital steward. It was in that role that he served at the First Battle of Manassas; he describes several cases of wounded soldiers whom he treated during and after that battle. Dr.

Thomas H. Williams arranged for Craighill to be examined by the Richmond Army Medical Board. He thought that the examination, which was oral, was devised to demonstrate the medical knowledge of the three examiners rather than the person being tested.

After a severe bout with pneumonia and diarrhea (diagnosed as typhoid-pneumonia), he was assigned to the small hospital at Gordonsville, Virginia, and later to the hospital center at Lynchburg. He treated many Federal prisoners. Just after the war, he was walking down the street in drab civilian clothes when he bumped into several Union soldiers who were part of the force occupying Lynchburg. They all "shook my hand with the greatest cordiality" and urged him to accept money and clothes from them, for they recognized him as their doctor when they had been prisoners. They regaled him with follow-up stories of soldiers upon whom he had operated and were now alive and well, though minus a limb, in Massachusetts.

Craven, John J. *Prison Life of Jefferson Davis.* New York: Carleton, 1866, 377 p. Reprinted as his *Fiction Distorting Fact.* With an introduction by Edward K. Eckert and annotations by Jefferson Davis. Macon, GA: Mercer University Press, 1987, 168 p.

Dr. Craven was the Union army physician assigned to examine and treat Jefferson Davis during the first seven months of his incarceration at Fortress Monroe. Davis suffered from severe pain in the head, diagnosed by Dr. Craven as a facial neuralgia, but more likely migraine headaches because of their throbbing nature and the accompanying visual change ("a cloud of black and amber motes rising and falling"). Jefferson Davis considered that the most inhumane action taken by the United States government during the War was to forbid the importation of quinine into the Confederacy. Some experts think that this work was not written by Craven, but by a political writer. This controversy is examined by Edward K. Eckert, who includes Jefferson Davis's own comments, taken from his personal copy of the book.

Crawford, Samuel W. *The History of the Fall of Fort Sumpter: The Genesis of the Civil War.* New York: F. P. Harper, 1887, 486 p. (Note: some printings have the primary and secondary titles reversed)

Crawford was the doctor with the Fort Sumter (often spelled Sumpter by contemporaries) garrison. A career army physician, he acted as a line officer and took charge of firing some batteries. He served as a combat officer during the remainder of the War and rose to the rank of brevet major general. This book is mainly about the political manueverings prior to secession, but also contains his personal description of the bombardment of Sumter. It contains no medical observations except a list of those killed and wounded during the bombardment and the ceremonial salute following the surrender.

Crocker, James F. "Prison Reminiscences." *Southern Historical Society Papers* 34 (1906): 28–51.

The author, a lieutenant, was taken prisoner during Pickett's charge at Gettyburg. He describes his wounding, his treatment by Federal surgeons, and his experiences as a prisoner. He had attended Pennsylvania College before the war and had friends in Gettysburg. Although a prisoner, he was allowed to leave the federal hospital and wander around Gettysburg. He visited the 11th Corps Hospital to see General Armistead, but he had died. He saw Armistead's grave and talked to his doctor, who, according to Crocker, attributed his death to the fact that "his proud spirit chafed under his imprisonment and his restlessness aggravated the wound."

The author was taken to the DeCamp Prison Hospital on David's Island in New York harbor. The wounded prisoners traveled by boat from Elizabethport because of the draft riot in Manhattan. Dr. James Simmons, the surgeon at DeCamp Hospital ordered all prisoners to discard their ragged uniforms, wash themselves, and wear only clean hospital clothing. The rags were burned. The prisoner-patients received "care and tenderness" from the Yankee doctors. They were visited by women from Manhattan, many of whom were openly Southern sympathizers.

Cullen, Thomas F. "Observations on the Influence of the Present War upon American Medicine and Surgery." *Medical Society of New Jersey Transactions* 98 (1864): 21–44.

In the annual essay for the New Jersey Medical Society, the author reviews how the war has changed medicine and surgery. New weapons are injuring more people in many ways. "Never before has the professional eye been directed to accidents so various and of such novel character as those now resulting in unprecedented numbers from the improved enginery of modern combat." He notes that the War, though fought between brothers, is bringing together "the once estranged sisters," medicine and surgery. He means that the surgeon sees the value of medical therapy in preventing epidemic diseases, while the medical doctor sees each day the value of surgery well-performed. The author describes the shock wave from large mortars, influencing not only the ears but also the entire nervous system. He states that the rifle and minie ball have such a tearing, whirling, splitting action that "their effects are more terrible" than previous round balls.

The author has many compaints about military medicine. He chastizes Surgeon General Hammond for his attempt to deprive his physicians of calomel and antimony, "the two most valuable levers in the treatment of disease." He criticizes a published report by Dr. John Swinburne, who amputated at the wrong time—during the height of inflammation—on a patient who had requested leave to return home and seek civilian surgical consultation. He is especially worried about the irregular practitioners who have become regimental surgeons and assistant surgeons. These individuals are not really doctors, he alleges, but members of "*one idea* sects" who represent "every wild *ism* born of half knowledge." Examining boards had removed most of these practitioners, but a few remain. After the war, the New Jersey Medical Society will have to change its rules to allow professional association with these practitioners, who, it is hoped, will have improved their medical knowledge during the War. In discussing these tests of medical ability, the author feels that many distinguished practitioners of good medicine did not appear before the medical board for fear that the questions would sample only book learning and not the wisdom gained by years of experience; the Board "placed their standard of literary knowledge in collateral branches far above the point attained by those whose attention has been chiefly devoted to the actual practice of medicine and surgery." One wonders if he is reporting his own experience.

Cupples, George. "Two Battle of Galveston Letters." Edited by Dorman H. Winfrey. *Southwestern Historical Quarterly* 65 (1961): 251–57.

George Cupples had been a doctor during the Mexican War and had later been president of the Texas Medical Association. In early 1863, he was the Confederate medical director of the District of Texas, New Mexico, and Arizona. On 1 January 1863, during the Battle of Galveston, he established the major support hospital in the Ursuline Convent; the nuns were helpful, mainly in obtaining food for the patients and staff. Many wounded soldiers arrived, brought by eight ambulance wagons. On the following day, Cupples received many Federal wounded, sailors from the *Harriet Lane* and soldiers from the 42nd Massachusetts. Federal physicians Ariel J. Cummings of the 42nd Massachusetts and naval surgeon Thomas A. Penrose treated the Federal prisoners, using Confederate stores. Cupples stated that relations between the Northern and

Southern physicians "are very agreeable." Union gunboats fired on the town and grapeshot hit the hospital. A piece of grapeshot struck Confederate surgeon S. A. W. Fischer (or Fisher) in the temple as he was tending to the wounded; the missle cut directly through his brain and exited the opposite temple, killing him instantly.

D

Da Costa, Jacob Mandes. *Medical Diagnosis.* Philadelphia: J. B. Lippincott, 1864, 694 p.

Da Costa produced this popular medical textbook during the War. He was an acting assistant surgeon in Philadelphia, first at the 16th and Filbert Hospital and later at Turner's Lane, where he supervised a ward for patients with heart disease. This textbook seldom mentions the War except to report a disease of the heart common in soldiers, characterized by palpitations, rapid heart beat, and a feeling of light headedness. In this work, Da Costa called the condition "irritable heart."

Dalton, John Call. *History of the College of Physicians and Surgeons in the City of New York: Medical Department of Columbia College.* New York: The College, 1888, 208 p.

Dalton was the premier academic physiologist in America during the War period. He never specifically mentions the War, but he does enumerate the faculty of the College of Physicians and Surgeons at various times. He mentions several individuals whose military careers were important. Edward Curtis, for example, graduated in medicine from the University of Pennsylvania in 1864; he immediately joined the Union army and was placed in charge of the microscopical section of the Army Medical Museum. He became a lecturer in histology at the College of Physicians and Surgeons in 1872 and professor of *materia medica* (pharmacology) in 1873.

Daniel, Ferdinand E. *Recollections of a Rebel Surgeon (and Other Sketches); or, In the Doctor's Sappy Says.* Austin, TX: Von Boeckmann, Schutze, and Company, 1899, 264 p.

The author, a surgeon with the hospitals of the Army of Tennessee, provides a few anecdotes written with humor. He was forced to improvise—to amputate using a pocket knife and a carpenter's saw. With a group of senior doctors present, including Foard, Stout, and Pim, the patient requested that Daniel, only twenty-four, perform a difficult operation (removal of the ends of bone broken through the skin). The author knew Frank Hawthorne, who had enlisted as a private with the 10th Alabama, but had ministered to a wounded soldier in the absence of doctors and was raised to the rank of assistant surgeon.

Dimon, Theodore. "A Federal Surgeon at Sharpsburg." Edited by James I. Robertson, Jr. *Civil War History* 6 (1960): 134–51.

At the Battle of Antietam, Dr. Theodore Dimon of the 2nd Maryland (Union) was detailed to organize a hospital in a red house and barn belonging to a farmer named J. F. Miller. In his diary and in a letter, he gives much detail about organizing the Miller Redhouse Hospital (as it was called) from scratch. On his own initiative, he grabbed stragglers. First he formed a guard of six men to keep order; the next group of stragglers he organized into five cooks and twelve nurses under his own hospital steward. He sent his black servant, Bob, to obtain food from army stores. Just over 140 wounded soldiers were assigned to him, and he placed them throughout the house and barn. He examined each, dressed the wound, noted those who needed operation, and set the time. "The minnie ball striking a bone," he told his wife, "does not permit much debate about amputation." He performed eleven limb amputations, one of which ended fatally with tetanus. He lost two other soldiers who had been shot through the lungs. When some of the stragglers whom he had pressed into duty were found consuming alcohol meant for the patients, he ordered the guards to string them up to apple trees by their thumbs, their toes just barely touching the ground. Within a week, he had evacuated about half the wounded to the general hospital in Frederick, Maryland.

"Dr. William A. Hammond, Surgeon General of the United States Army." *Harper's Weekly* (21 November 1863): 748.

A short but detailed review of Hammond's prewar career states that he apprenticed medicine under Dr. E. N. Roberts of Harrisburg at age sixteen. After graduation from the University of New York, he served at the Pennsylvania Hospital before joining the United States Army on 29 June 1849. Three years of "Indian wars" at Santa Fe, New Mexico, "brought on a functional disorder of the heart." After service in Florida, at West Point, and at Fort Riley (four years), his disordered constitution required a trip to Europe to restore his health. Upon his return, he spent a year at Fort Mackinaw before going as a civilian to the University of Maryland. The source of this information is not stated but must have been based on an interview with Hammond. A woodcut shows Hammond in his best form.

Douglas, J. H., and C. W. Brink. *Reports on the Operations of the Inspectors and Relief Agents of the Sanitary Commission after the Battle of Fredericksburg, December 13, 1862.* New York: W. C. Bryant, 1863, 31 p.

This brief report gives the location and activities of each Union field hospital at the Battle of Fredericksburg. It lists the doctors in charge and the operators and gives casualty figures. Specific criticisms of each hospital are included; for example, the 1st Division Hospital: "Supplies were not sufficient. Soft bread and fresh beef were not served." The report includes a copy of Letterman's orders before the battle.

E

Edmonds, S. Emma E. *The Female Spy of the Union Army.* Boston: DeWolfe, Fisk, and Co., 1864, 384 p. Reprinted as her *Nurse and Spy in the Union Army,* Illustrated with woodcuts. Hartford, CT: W. S. Williams, 1865, 384 p.

Although full of improbable adventures, this book describes some aspects of hospital life that may be accurate. The author claims to have been present at First Manassas. Two hundred pages describe the author's adventures during the Peninsula campaign. According to the book, the author was present during the Battle of Antietam and the siege of Vicksburg.

Ellis, Thomas T. *Leaves from the Diary of an Army Surgeon; or Incidents of Field Camp and Hospital Life.* New York: John Bradburn, 1863, 312 p.

While this work is mainly a description of the military activities of the Army of the Potomac from the Peninsula campaign through Second Bull Run to Antietam, the author includes several very interesting eyewitness observations of his own. Ellis quite vividly describes the Federal supply center on the Pamunkey called the White House. The only building within sight was the home that gave the place its name, formerly the residence of Martha Custis before she became Mrs. George Washington. Many wounded were present, and many hospital ships were in the river, but, according to Ellis, no one had taken authority to begin the evacuation. Ellis later describes the burning of White House, the wounded left behind at Savage Station, the hospitals at Fortress Monroe, and the

Union doctor Thomas Ellis wrote about his medical experiences during the Peninsula campaign of 1862 while the War was still being fought. In this letter, George Brinton McClellan, the commander of Union forces on the Peninsula, gives Ellis permission to dedicate the book to him.

evacuation from Harrison's Landing on the James River. Ellis was later present on the battlefield under flag of truce after Second Bull Run. His description of Antietam is less detailed. Published during the war, this book is dedicated to General McClellan.

Elmore, A. M. "Some Recollections of the Medical Officers of the Indian Territory, C.S.A." *Southern Practitioner* 25 (1903): 706–8.

The author began the War as a private with the 29th Texas Cavalry. The regimental doctors were named Kearby, Rochelle, and R. W. Reed, who practiced in Texarkana after the war. The author became a dispensary steward at the North Fork General Hospital in Indian Territory. The surgeon-in-charge was named Evans; his assistants, both from Missouri, were named Lee and Alexander. Toward the end of the War, Indian regiments were formed. The First Choctaw and Chickasaw Infantry Regiment had W. J. Crowdus as surgeon. The author became assistant surgeon of the regiment despite his lack of medical training. The Second Choctaw and Chickasaw Infantry Regiment had a surgeon named Turner; the position of assistant surgeon went unfilled.

Eve, Paul F. *A Collection of Remarkable Cases in Surgery.* Philadelphia: J. B. Lippincott, 1857, 858 p.

Eve was a leading Southern surgeon, president of the American Medical Association in 1857–58. This book of his most interesting cases, according to Rutkow, "provides some of the most enjoyable and entertaining reading to be found in any nineteenth-century American surgical text." Eve had military medical experience as a volunteer in European wars; for example, he treated the wounded during the Austro-Italian War of 1859. During the Civil War, Eve was the surgeon general of the State of Tennessee, but spent most of the War in charge of the Gate City Hospital in Atlanta.

Eve, Paul F. "Report of Eight Cases of Lithotomy Peformed during the War." *Nashville Journal of Medicine and Surgery* 1 (1866): 136.

This report describes an interesting patient, referred to only as "Mr. O'B.," whose case demonstrated the danger of infection in a military hospital. Dr. Eve performed lithotomy for bladder stone upon this patient in 1849; this was repeated by a different surgeon in 1854. In April 1863, the patient, then fifty-six, again consulted Eve about recurrence of bladder stone. Eve performed a third operation upon this civilian in a military hospital, Gate City Hospital, Atlanta. On the twelfth postoperative day, an infection developed on the wrist, where no wound had been known to exist. This spread to erysipelas of the entire arm, leading to amputation and death.

F

Farris, John Kennerly. "A Confederate Surgeon's View of Fort Donelson: The Diary of John Kennerly Farris." Edited by Jim Stanbery. *Civil War Regiments: A Journal of the American Civil War* 1 (1991): 7–19.

The author was hospital steward of the 41st Tennessee. This selection from his diary and the editor's comments emphasize the military aspects of the defense of Fort Donelson, but a few medical observations are included.

Fisk, Wilbur. *Anti-Rebel: The Civil War Letters of Wilbur Fisk.* Croton-on-Hudson, NY: Emil Rosenblatt, 1983, 361 p.

During the War, Private Wilbur Fisk regularly submitted letters to the *Green Mountain Freeman* of Vermont. Of special medical interest is Fisk's service as a hospital guard with the 6th Corps Hospital at City Point, Virginia, in the last few months of the War. He describes a typical hospital tent—actually three tents sewn together. Each of the three parts contained six beds, three on a side, with a space between beds almost as large as the bed itself. Each bed consisted of an iron bedstead, a cloth tick filled with straw for a mattress, and plenty of blankets. On 2 February 1865, all the hospitals at City Point received a sudden injection of a large number of sick as the troops along the Petersburg front prepared to march. Throughout the evening, Fisk and other guards had to clean out a wooden shack that had been used as a carpenter's shop. Material was just thrown out of the windows as the building was made ready to accept fifty sick men.

Fitch, Charles. "Dr. Fitch's Report on the Fort Pillow Massacre." Edited by John Cimprich and Robert C. Mainfort. *Tennessee Historical Quarterly* 44 (1985): 27–39.

Dr. Fitch was a contract surgeon assigned to the 13th Tennessee Cavalry (Union). He was in Fort Pillow when it was taken by troops under Nathan Bedford Forrest on 12 April 1864. This official eye-witness report was written on 30 April and long lost in the "Returns of Medical Officers," Record Group 94, National Archives. Dr. Fitch tried to treat the wounded, but was kept under guard for his own protection, by the direct order of General Forrest. He saw many black soldiers shot to death long after the surrender.

"Foreign Correspondence: America." *Medical Times and Gazette* (London) 1 (1865): 127–29, 153–54.

An anonymous medical observer from a London medical journal observed Union medical facilities near Petersburg, Virginia, writing this report on 28 December 1864. The description of events is quite romantic. He states that these medical officers received brevet promotions for meritorious service: A. McParlen [actually Thomas A. McParlin], medical director, Army of the Potomac; Alexander N. Dougherty, medical director, 2nd Corps; J. J. Milhaw, medical director, 5th Corps; and Charles Smart, medical inspector, 2nd Corps.

Formento, Felix, Jr. *Louisiana Soldier's Relief Association and Hospital in the City of Richmond, Virginia.* Richmond, VA: Tyler, Wise, Allegre, and Smith, 1862, 38 p.

The Louisiana Hospital of Richmond was located about one mile from the city in buildings that had been the Baptist College. The main building of the former college was three stories and held 300 beds. A surgeon on duty slept in the building each night to handle emergencies. A separate building housed the wounded and sick officers. Nurses consisted of eight Sisters of Charity and twelve enlisted men (two of whom remained at Manassas to aid the evacuation of Louisiana soldiers). The Confederate government gave the hospital twenty-two cents per day per soldier as commutations of rations plus paying the salaries of the enlisted nurses. The rest of the cost of the hospital was paid by donations from Louisiana handled by the Relief Association (a financial report by John Perkins, Jr. is included). In the last three months of 1861, the hospital admitted 824 patients, of whom 477 returned to duty, 117 were discharged from the army by medical disability, and 47 died and were buried in Hollywood Cemetery. The report gives the names, diagnoses, and dispositions of each of the 824 admissions.

Formento, Felix Jr. *Notes and Observations on Army Surgery.* New Orleans: L. E. Marchand, 1863. Reprint. San Francisco: Norman Publishing, 1990, 62 pages.

The author was born in New Orleans, but received his medical training in Europe. He was present at the battles of Solferino and Magenta in Sardinia in 1859. He returned to New Orleans in 1860 and, during the War, organized and directed the Louisiana Hospital in Richmond. He returned to New Orleans, now occupied by Federal troops, in 1863 and wrote the present pamphlet. It concerns his military medical experiences in Sardinia and in Richmond. He attributed the low death rate at the Louisiana Hospital, calculated by him as 11.9 per 1,000 admissions, to the dedicated service of Catholic nuns from New Orleans. He removed patients with cellulitis (called by him erysipelas) or gangrene from the main hospital building and placed them in tents on the grounds where the ventilation was better. Formento describes the serious smallpox epidemic that began in September of 1862.

Forman, Jacob G. *The Western Sanitary Commission.* St. Louis: R. P. Studley, 1864, 144 p.

This book describes the origin and working of the Western Sanitary Commission, an organization formed in St. Louis on the model of the United States Sanitary Commission. The president of the

Commission, James E. Yeatman, accompanied a fleet of vessels to the battlefield at Shiloh; many of these, including the *City of Louisiana,* the *D. A. January,* the *Imperial,* and the *Empress,* had been outfitted by the funds of the Western Commission. The Western Sanitary Commission inspected military general hospitals and awarded cash prizes to the enlisted men and nurses of the cleanest ones.

Foster, John Y. "Four Days at Gettysburg." *Civil War Times Illustrated* 11 (April 1972): 19–23.

After hearing about the Battle of Gettysburg, the Ascension Church in Philadelphia sent supplies to the Christian Commission on the battlefield. The author accompanied those supplies and gives a riveting description of medical treatment at Camp Letterman on or about 11 July. Most of the supplies were given to the rebels, who needed them more. Rebel surgeons had turned a large barn into a makeshift hospital with wounded on the floor packed so solidly that it was "almost impossible for one to stir without communicating the shock to all." In the center of the barn, Confederate surgeons were operating and "there, in full view of hundreds of enfeebled wretches, the process of cutting, and carving, and butchering (for it was nothing else) went on day after day." Foster was angered that the wounded were "compulsory witnesses of the atrocities which these surgeons dignified by the name of operations." The rebels, both wounded and doctors, were at first surprised, and then very grateful, upon receiving food and supplies from the Christian Commission.

Freeman, Douglas Southall. "Papers Relating to the Medical Department of the Confederate States Army." In his *A Calendar of Confederate Papers,* pp. 15–50. Richmond, VA: Whittiet and Shepperson, 1908.

This work summarizes all the medical manuscripts in the Confederate Museum in Richmond. All of the correspondence relating to the military hospital in Front Royal, Virginia, later moved to Liberty, Virginia, is reproduced. The medical director of the Army of the Potomac, Thomas H. Williams, authorized the surgeon-in-charge of Front Royal Hospital to "press free negroes into service" to act as nurses, relieving enlisted men of nursing duties to allow them to return to military commands. The papers also contain excerpts from the minutes of the Association of Army and Navy Surgeons of the Confederate States, organized in 1863. The Museum also contains the original register of admissions to the Robertson Hospital in Richmond; Freeman summarizes the 1,333 admissions, with 73 deaths, and lists the women who supported the hospital and the doctors who worked there.

G

Gaillard, Edwin S. *The Medical and Surgical Lessons of the Late War.* Louisville, KY: Louisville Journal Job Print, 1868, 16 p.

The author was a Confederate surgeon and observed Confederate medicine, he says, from northern Virginia to Mississippi. The surgical lessons were: (1) contrary to the statement of Macleod from the Crimea, trephination can be of value in the treatment of depressed skull fracture and even, occasionally, in treating idiocy and epilepsy resulting from head trauma; (2) again contrary to Macleod, amputation at the hip is not always fatal; and (3) good ventilation prevents the wound complications of tetanus and gangrene. Gaillard credits H. F. Campbell with devising the treatment of hospital gangrene by litigating the major artery of the affected limb. The medical lessons of the war were: (1) quinine prevents malaria; (2) yellow fever (except perhaps in south Texas) is not endemic, but comes in by ship and, as shown by the Federal experience in New Orleans, can be prevented by tight quarantine; (3) the use of the lancet to induce bleeding is of no benefit in any condition; (4) measles and other diseases are self-limited and need no special treatment; and (5) the blockade showed most medicines and tonics that had been taken by the populace before the War to sustain health were worthless. It is Gaillard's opinion that the large ulcers resulting from vaccination were due to the poor general health of the soldiers (mainly from dietary deficiency) and not from infected vaccine.

Galloupe, Isaac F. "Medical history of the Seventeenth Regiment Mass. Volunteers." *Boston Medical and Surgical Journal* 68 (1863): 136–41.

After being crowded together aboard ship, twenty-five soldiers of the 17th Massachusetts developed typhoid fever; five died. After arrival at New Bern, North Carolina, the biggest problem was malaria. "The Regiment having been much exposed to night air, suffered extremely from such exposure; nearly every man in the Regiment having had at least once an attack of miasmatic disease. In the month of August, 1,100 cases are reported (in a regiment of less than 900). The Regiment became so much reduced as to be hardly able to perform camp guard duty." Only three fatalities occurred due to malaria, but, in some soldiers, "the constitution was completely broken down, and the men were discharged from service." Quinine was effective in treating established cases but had no value in prophylaxis; "companies which took these medicines daily appeared to be as much affected by the disease as those who did not take it." This letter, dated 20 February 1863, gives regimental statistics. Beginning with 842 men, 252 replacements were received. The regiment suffered the deaths of two men in combat and three by drowning. A total of 161 had been discharged for medical reasons.

Galloupe, Isaac F. "Cerebro-spinal Affection." *Boston Medical and Surgical Journal* 68 (1863): 203–6.

In this letter from New Bern, North Carolina, written 20 March 1863, Galloupe describes a terrible epidemic that killed five men in the 45th Massachusetts, seventeen in the 51st Massachusetts, and one civilian, the nine-year-old son of an officer. The local civilian physician reported he had never seen anything like this. The patient experienced pain in the head, back, and legs followed by vomiting, delirium, sometimes petechiae, and, in every case but one, death. Autopsy showed inflammation of the meningeal covering of the brain and spinal cord. [This was certainly meningococcal meningitis.]

The author adds observations about treating wounds. He favors early operation, even comparing similar wounds treated by amputation or by simple dressing. In those instances where the author tried to save the limb by simple dressing, the "patient finally lost his limb, and in some cases his life also." Galloupe compares combat injuries with similar civilian injuries. "The severe shock and depression of spirits which immediately follow severe wounds in civil life, do not often appear in those injured in battle, unless some vital organ is injured and the wound is mortal. On the contrary, the patients are in a high state of excitement and exhiliration."

Gammage, Washington L. *The Camp, the Bivouac, and the Battlefield, Being a History of the Fourth Arkansas Regiment.* Selma, AL: Cooper and Kimball, 1864, 164 p.

Gammage was surgeon of the 4th Arkansas, present at the battles of Pea Ridge, Stone's River, and Chickamauga. The work is of special interest because it was published in the Confederacy. It is basically a regimental history that just happens to be written by the regimental surgeon. The assistant surgeon of the regiment was F. N. Jones. The hospital steward, Dr. E. W. Kerr of Hempstead County, was a private who was a doctor. One of the few medical observations made by Gammage concerns the huge epidemic of measles that occurred when the regiment was stationed at Mount Vernon, Arkansas in 1861; thirty soldiers died despite being nursed by local women volunteers.

Gildersleeve, John R. "Chimborazo Hospital during 1861–1865." *Confederate Veteran* 12 (1904): 577–79. Reprinted as his "History of Chimborazo Hospital, C.S.A." *Southern Historical Society Papers* 36 (1908): 86–94.

The author states that during the War, Chimborazo admitted 76,000 soldiers, of whom 17,000 were wounded; the death rate was 9 percent. Dr. Gildersleeve began service with the Midway Hospital in Charlottesville under James Cabell. He spent the middle years of the War at Chimborazo and the last year with the 20th South Carolina of Kershaw's Brigade.

Gill, John C. "An Ohio Doctor Views Campaigning on the White River, 1864." Edited by Harry F. Lupold. *Arkansas Historical Quarterly* 34 (1975): 333–51.

Born in 1836, Dr. Gill graduated from Western Reserve Medical School in 1859. He was assistant surgeon of the 120th Ohio during the White River campaign of September 1864. His regiment was healthy at the start of the campaign, with only three soldiers excused from duty. He noted that the water of the White River "is clear as crystal yet there is something in it that induces diarrhea."

Gill, John C. "A Union Surgeon Views the War from Kentucky, 1862." Edited by Harry F. Lupold. *Register of the Kentucky Historical Society* 72 (1974): 272–75.

When he wrote this letter on 2 March 1862, Dr. Gill was assistant surgeon of the 65th Ohio. He stayed behind in Stanford, Kentucky, south of Lexington, to treat seven soldiers with typhoid fever while his clothes and money went on with his regiment. He cleared out a church, put straw on the floor, and used blankets for beds. Two soliders died: "they were delirious, tongues like a burnt piece of leather." The other five survived, and Dr. Gill was "gratified with the result." After the War, he practiced medicine in Cleveland, Ohio, dying in 1921.

Goldsmith, Middleton. *A Report on Hospital Gangrene, Erysipelas, and Pyemia, as Observed in the Department of the Ohio and the Cumberland, with Cases Appended.* Louisville, KY: Bradley and Gilbert, 1863, 94 p.

Goldsmith is usually credited with devising the bromine treatment of hospital gangrene. He states that he first got the idea when he read that Dr. Brainard of Chicago, experimenting with the effects of snakebite, note that the gangrenous aspects of the bite were decreased if the poison were mixed with iodine. Dr. Goldsmith used a different halogen, bromine, because iodine was difficult to handle chemically. His bromine application procedure began with the scraping of the surface of the gangrenous lesion until nothing remained but a bleeding, soft, flocculent pulp. This scraping was so painful that the wounded man usually had to be anesthetized. When the bleeding stopped, bromine was painted over the entire surface, coagulating the soft pulp. Two of the first four experimental subjects were captured Confederates. All four had been wounded in the Battle of Stone's River and had arrived at the Federal hospital in Louisville about 15 January 1863. All four of these soldiers survived. Of a larger number treated with bromine, only 3 percent died; of a previous, smaller group not treated with bromine, 50 percent died.

Grace, William. *The Army Surgeon's Manual.* New York: Balliere Brothers, 1864, 200 p. 2d edition, enlarged. New York: Balliere Brothers, 1865, 225 p. Reprint. San Francisco: Norman Publishing, 1991, 200 p.

This manual contains the rules and regulations of the United States Army Medical Department, all general orders of the War Department, and all circulars from the Surgeon General's Office up to 1 July 1864. It also lists the medical staff of the regular army as of 1 July 1864. [I was unable to examine this work.]

Greenleaf, Charles R. *A Manual for the Medical Officers of the United States Army.* Philadelphia: J. B. Lippincott, 1864, 199 p.

This brief medical manual describes the duties of the medical officer and provides blank forms that the officer fills out monthly. Separate chapters describe the duties of medical inspectors, medical directors, medical purveyors, staff surgeons, and contract surgeons.

Gross, Samuel D. *A Manual of Military Surgery; or Hints on the Emergencies of Field, Camp and Hospital Practice.* Philadelphia: J. B. Lippincott, 1861. Reprint. San Francisco: Norman Publishing, 1988, 186 p.

Gross held the chair of surgery at Jefferson Medical College and was probably the greatest practicing surgeon in America. He adapted his manual from a medical article, writing it in nine days. He recommended conservative surgery; just as the surgeon tries to save a man's life, so should he also try to save his limb. The Confederacy published the work in Richmond. It was translated into Japanese in 1874.

Grosvenor, Charles H. "Letter." *Cincinnati Gazette,* 31 October 1862.

The author accompanied Lieutenant David B. Carlin of the 18th Ohio, who had been severely wounded at Chickamauga, in an attempt to travel to Cincinnati overland. On the 24th of October, as Grosvenor "came down the cheerless and horribly muddy road leading down the valley of Sequatchie from Chattanooga to Stevenson, I saw on the riverbank three or four hospital tents." Riding up, they saw a placard reading "Soldier's Home" and were met by the chaplain of the 101st Ohio, who had been detailed to act as an agent of the United States Sanitary Commission. His food and his cheer made their further evacuation possible. [Carlin was discharged on 4 June 1864, and Grosvenor transferred to a veteran regiment on 20 October 1864.]

H

Habersham, S. E. "Observations upon the Statistics of Chimborazo Hospital, with Remarks upon the Treatment of Various Diseases during the Recent Civil War." *Nashville Journal of Medicine and Surgery* 1 (1866): 416–28.

Habersham was a Confederate army surgeon with the 2nd Division of Chimborazo Hospital. He stayed behind and surrendered the hospital to Federal forces after the fall of Richmond. "Through the courtesy of Surgeon Stone, U.S.A.," he copied the total hospital statistics from when it opened in 10 October 1861 to 1 November 1863. He states that the pavilion system on the Chimborazo hills east of Richmond were originally built as winter quarters for the Army of Northern Virginia. When the Army remained near Manassas during the winter of 1861–62, Surgeon General S. P. Moore, "with the promptness that characterized all of his executive acts," took over the buildings for a huge hospital to house the great number of wounded and, especially, the sick. He describes the size, heating, and ventilation of wards and discusses several of the major diseases such as typhoid fever and hospital gangrene. His major medical method involved changing the internal balance of the sick patient; he decried the lack of available stimulants, especially brandy.

Haddaway, Claude Lee. "With Loyalty and Honor as a Patriot:

Recollections of a Confederate Soldier." Edited by Royce Shingleton. *Alabama Historical Quarterly* 33 (1971): 240–63.

Hadaway enlisted in the 22nd Alabama in August of 1861 at age sixteen. He wrote this memoir of his service in 1933. He was present at the battles of Shiloh, Vicksburg, Atlanta, Franklin, and Nashville, but the major medical observations of his military career concern his illness at Corinth, Mississippi, in June 1862. He developed "typhoid pneumonia" and was evacuated by boxcar. The train did not move for three hours, and it was so hot that he climbed upon the boxcar roof. The train pulled out, and he rode atop his car to Columbus, Mississippi. He was taken to a tent not far from a stream. There were three sick in each tent, and the soldiers on either side of him died. No one would give him water, so he crawled down to the stream on his own. A friend finally found him and helped him get enough to eat. He attributed his survival to "a perfect constitution and an invincible will." His greatest enemies during this period were "hunger and the doctors."

Hamilton, Frank H. *A Practical Treatise on Fractures and Dislocations*. Philadelphia: Blanchard and Lea, 1860. Reprint. San Francisco: Norman Publishing, 1991, 757 p.

Hamilton was a leading American surgeon, having graduated from the University of Pennsylvania in 1833. According to Rutkow, this is the first American text to deal in depth with fractures. The first edition appeared just before the War; other editions followed regularly. The 6th edition of 1880 had grown to 909 pages.

Hamilton, Frank H. *A Practical Treatise on Military Surgery*. New York: Balliere Brothers, 1861. Reprint. San Francisco: Norman Publishing, 1989, 234 p.

This book was written by a well-known New York surgeon after he had had military medical experience as surgeon of the 33rd New York at First Bull Run. There are separate chapters on all aspects of military medicine including examination of recruits, hygiene, hospitals, conveyance (evacuation), gunshot wounds, amputations, diarrhea, hospital gangrene, and scurvy. Hamilton quotes the United States Army 1860 study of ambulances and includes the 1861 United States Army medical regulations in an appendix.

Hamilton, Frank H. *A Treatise on Military Surgery and Hygiene*. New York: Bailliere Brothers, 1865, 648 p.

Hamilton wrote this work after he had served as medical inspector with the Army of the Potomac. He dedicated it to Major General E. D. Keyes, who had commanded the 4th Corps during the Peninsula campaign (but who had resigned from the army and was a civilian when the book was written). The work contains chapters on the examination of recruits, on hygiene, on hospitals, and on preparations for the field. These are followed by chapters on the treatment of gunshot wounds in various portions of the body, the treatment of arrow wounds, specific operations such as amputation and exsection, and on diseases such as gangrene, tetanus, and scurvy.

The author is obviously writing from a vast personal experience. When he examines the effects of gunshot wounds of the heart, he describes an execution he attended where the deserter received such wounds under his direct observation. He reports specific wounds in specific soldiers. He shares the experiences of other army physicians, from both published reports and conversation. He quotes a letter from Dr. Hachenberg to the Surgeon General recommending turpentine to prevent the spread of hospital gangrene. Rutkow considers this book a second edition of Hamilton's *Practical Treatise on Military Surgery,* but it is based upon a much larger experience described in much greater detail.

Hammond, William A. "On Uraemic Intoxication." *American Journal of the Medical Sciences* 41 (1861): 55–83.

Hammond created renal failure in dogs by experimental surgery. He anesthetized dogs with chloroform, then removed both kidneys. The dog without kidneys could survive only a few days; he had ammonia on his exhaled breath. This article shows the type of research interest that Hammond had when he was Professor of Anatomy and Physiology at the University of Maryland, just before he rejoined the army.

Hammond, William A. "Annual Report of the Surgeon-General, U.S.A." *Boston Medical and Surgical Journal* 67 (1863): 437–43.

Hammond's official report for fiscal year 1862 includes expenditures and a complete list of all 150 general hospitals, with the number of patients in each one, totalling 58,715, on 30 June 1862.

Hammond, William A. "Circular to the Medical Profession." *Boston Medical and Surgical Journal* 68 (1863): 108–9.

In this circular, reprinted in many medical journals, Hammond reiterates his intention to prepare a surgical history of the rebellion. He asks every physician, civilian or military, who treats a soldier wounded in service to send his observations to the Surgeon General's Office. His growing interest in neurology is indicated by his special paragraph which reads: "In those patients in whom injuries of the skull have occurred, or upon whom the trephine has been applied, the mental and physical conditions should alike be dwelt upon."

Hammond, William A. *A Treatise on Hygiene, with Special Reference to the Military Service.* Philadelphia: J. B. Lippincott, 1863. Reprint. San Francisco: Norman Publishing, 1991, 604 p.

This work presents Hammond's ideas on military medicine. It includes floor plans on all the major hospitals of the world, telling what is good and what is bad about each one. He is most critical of the hospital built by his predecessor at Hilton Head, South Carolina (p. 312). Hammond gives his opinion that blacks will never make good soldiers, but then adds a note in proof (presumably after some personal experiences to change his mind) that this opinion may have been in error.

Hammond, William A., ed. *Military Medical and Surgical Essays.* Philadelphia: J. B. Lippincott, 1864, 522 p.

Most of these essays were printed as pamphlets and distributed to medical officers early in the war by the United States Sanitary Commission. This collection includes essays by William H. Van Buren on quinine (a scholarly historical review proving its value in treating and in preventing malaria), by Elisha Harris on epidemic diseases, by Austin Flint on pneumonia, by Stephen Smith on amputation, by Valentine Mott on how to stop bleeding, by Richard Hodges on excision of joints, and by the editor on scurvy.

Hammond, William A. *A Statement of the Causes Which Led to the Dismissal of Surgeon-General William A. Hammond from the Army, with a Review of the Evidence Adduced before the Court.* Washington, DC: privately printed, 1864, 73 p.

Hammond prepared this detailed refutation of the charge against him. He concludes that he, "conscious of right, will patiently wait for the full vindication which is sure to come."

Hancock, Cornelia. *South after Gettysburg: Letters of Cornelia Hancock, 1863–1868.* Edited by Henrietta S. Jaquette. New York: Thomas Y. Crowell, 1937, 288 p.

Dr. Henry T. Child of the Union army asked his sister-in-law to come to the Gettysburg battlefield on 5 July to help with the wounded. She was a nurse at Camp Letterman from 6 July to 31 August. She served at City Point hospitals during the campaign of 1864.

Hard, Abner. *History of the Eighth Cavalry Regiment, Illinois Volunteers, during the Great Rebellion.* Aurora, IL: privately printed, 1868. Reprint. Dayton, OH: Morningside Press, 1984, 368 p.

The author was surgeon of the 8th Illinois Cavalry, but his narrative concentrate on military rather than medical activities. The regiment served with the Army of the Potomac during most of the war, being heavily engaged at Gettysburg (supposedly firing the first shot). During the last few months of the war, the regiment garrisoned northern Virginia, often opposing Mosby's raiders.

Harrison, Samuel A. "The Civil War Journal of Dr. Samuel A. Harrison." Edited by Charles L. Wagandt. *Civil War History* 13 (1967): 131–46.

Samuel A. Harrison was a civilian doctor who practiced in Maryland throughout the War. His journal contains much information on political issues, especialiy emancipation in Maryland, but Dr. Harrison has virtually no comments of a medical nature.

Hart, Albert Gaillard. "The Surgeon and the Hospital in the Civil War." *Military Historical Society of Massachusetts Papers* 13 (1913): 229–86.

The author was surgeon of the 41st Ohio and was present at the Battles of Murfreesboro, Chickamauga, and Missionary Ridge. He took part in the amphibious operation at Brown's Ferry. During the Georgia campaign, Dr. Hart was assigned to the general hospital of the Army of the Cumberland. He and about twelve other doctors were treating 600 patients in the tent hospital when they were overwhelmed by the sudden arrival of 1,200 additional casualties from the Battle of Kennesaw Mountain.

Hawkes, Esther Hill. *A Woman Doctor's Civil War: Esther Hill Hawkes' Diary.* Edited by Gerald Schwartz. Columbia: University of South Carolina Press, 1984, 301 p.

Hawkes graduated from the New England Female Medical College in 1857. During the Civil War, she served as a civilian physician on the South Carolina Sea Islands, generally ministering to black refugees.

Hilgard, Eugene. "A Confederate Scientist at War." Edited by Walter E. Pittman. *Civil War Times Illustrated* 25 (March 1986): 20.

Eugene Hilgard was a leading chemist and geologist in nineteenth-century America. He was the state geologist of Mississippi and on the faculty of the University in Oxford when the War began. He used his chemical knowledge to help build oxygen-hydrogen searchlights on the Vicksburg bluffs to illuminate Union vessels. He developed a severe case of dysentery and was a patient at the military hospital in Jackson when the Federals under Grant temporarily took the town; they examined the hospital, but did not interfere with the medical work. Later, Hilgard acted as a nurse at the hospital in Oxford that occupied many of the university's buildings. "I took charge of about a dozen wounded," he writes. "who at first rebelled at the idea of a non-medical man dressing their wounds." But later, the wounded told Hilgard that "I was more tender with them than the doctor and hurt them less." Hilgard spent much of his life after the War on the faculty of the University of California, Berkeley, where he helped found the scientific study of soils.

Hodges, Richard M. *The Excision of Joints.* Cambridge, MA: Welch and Bigelow, 1861, 204 p.

Hodges was an 1850 graduate of the medical department of Harvard University. He practiced surgery at the Massachusetts General Hospital. This work concerns the operation to remove joints damaged by gunshot wounds while saving the limb. The limb postoperatively is shortened but retains significant function. Hodges wrote a pamphlet on this topic published by the United States Sanitary Commission and reproduced in *Medical and Surgical Essays,* edited by Hammond.

Holden, Edgar. "The First Cruise of the Monitor *Passaic.*" *Harper's New Monthly Magazine* 156 (1863): 577–95.

The author was the naval surgeon on the U.S.S. *Passaic.* In its maiden voyage from New York to the sea islands off South Carolina, the *Passaic* passed through the same storm off Cape Hatteras that sank the original *Monitor.* The article describes the unsuccessful attack of the *Passaic* and other ships upon the harbor defenses of Charleston ("30 guns against 400"), but contains no medical observations whatsoever. In fact, the article does not identify the author as a doctor.

Holmes, Oliver Wendell. "My Hunt after the Captain." *Atlantic Monthly* 10 (1862): 738–64.

Holmes was a leading physician of the Civil War era and a nationally famous writer. He was awakened one night by the delivery of a telegram that notified him that his son had been shot through the neck, but the wound was "thought not mortal." All he could think about was the long list of important structures that ran through the neck: the trachea, the esophagus, the carotid arteries, the jugular veins. He set off the next day to try to find his son. On the way, he saw some of the wounded from the Battle of Antietam: "a pitiable sight, truly pitiable, yet so vast, so far beyond the possibility of relief." The account is interesting for his interviews with many people, civilian and military, Union soldier and rebel prisoner, but contains few medical observations.

Holstein, Anna Morris. *Three Years in Field Hospitals of the Army of the Potomac.* Philadelphia: J. B. Lippincott, 1867, 131 p.

The author, identified on the title page only as "Mrs. H.," was a volunteer nurse with the 2nd Corps, Army of the Potomac. She was present at the Battle of Antietam. She arrived at Gettysburg about a week after the battle and took charge of the 2nd Corps diet kitchen, a part of Camp Letterman. She thought that the medical care was superior at the battle of Gettysburg; "there was no long-continued suffering as in the earlier battles of the war." She recounts how a young soldier, Luther White, was believed dead. His burial was ordered, but, just before he was lowered into a grave, he roused and asked the burial detail, "Boys, what are you doing?" After a surprised exchange, he looked into the grave, which already contained one body and said, "I won't be buried by this raw recruit." He continued to improve and was evacuated to Chestnut Hill Hospital, Philadelphia where he wrote Holstein, telling her that the doctors there predicted his survival. By 7 August, only 3,000 wounded remained around Gettysburg and they were all moved to Camp Letterman on the York turnpike. She heard President Lincoln's address.

Howard, Benjamin. "Treatment of Gun-shot Wounds of Chest and Abdomen." *Boston Medical and Surgical Journal* 69 (1863–64): 42–43.

Although holding the rank of assistant surgeon, United States Army, the author reports himself as surgeon-in-chief, artillery brigade, 5th Corps. He has devised a new dressing to maintain the integrity of the thorax or abdomen opened by a bullet wound. After bleeding ceases, he brings the edges of the wound as close together as he can, then puts metallic sutures through them to maintain this position. The remaining hole he covers with shreds of charpie hardened by collodion. "The natural condition of the parts is now approximately restored. The lung is suspended in a closed cavity; the volume of air admitted while the wound was open soon becomes absorbed, and the lung is again at liberty to expand freely.

The most distressing symptom, *dyspnea,* is relieved immediately."
He reports two successful administrations of this dressing in soldiers wounded at the Battle of Chancellorsville.

Howard, E. Lloyd. "The Effects of Minie Balls on Bone." *Confederate Medical and Surgical Journal* 1 (1864): 88–89.

Wounds produced by the minie ball "are characterized by extensive fissuring and comminution, such as was rarely, if ever, seen when the old smooth-bore musket was the weapon of the soldier." The author attempts to use physical principles to explain why the new bullet produces such splintering of bone.

Hubbard, George H. "Spurious Vaccination: Inoculation with Virus Supposed to be Syphilitic." *Medical and Surgical Reporter* 14 (1866): 103.

In November of 1863, the author arrived at Fort Smith, Arkansas, to take assignment as medical director of the Army of the Frontier. He encountered several hundred soldiers who had developed inflammation at the site of smallpox inoculation. The first day, they developed a severe itch, the next day yellow pustules occurred in the inoculation area; these increased in size until they burst, leaving a large open ulcer with an unpleasant discharge. This condition was followed by fever and by swelling of the glands in the armpit. He investigated this problem, concluding that "the virus which caused all these cases came from persons who had been vaccinated in the rebel army." The disease was brought to Fort Smith by rebel deserters and by Union soldiers who had been vaccinated—sometimes against their will—while rebel prisoners. It was then spread to other Union soldiers by "ignorant medical officers" and by troops practicing self-inoculation. Six soldiers "vaccinated" by this method later came down with smallpox, showing that the "virus" that was inoculated was not the smallpox virus. The author concludes that the material being passed from soldier to soldier was syphilis.

"The Hypodermic Syringe: First Used in Confederate States Army." *Southern Historical Society Papers* 31 (1903): 372.

This article reprints (but does not give the author of) a brief item from the *Chattanooga News* of 10 February 1904 (the *Southern Historical Society Papers* appeared after their imprint date). The unidentified author used a hypodermic syringe at Ringgold, Georgia, during late 1863 or early 1864. He obtained it from a civilian colleague, J. P. K. Walker of Augusta. No physician with the Army of Tennessee had ever seen one. The author relieved pain by injecting morphine into the back.

I

Imboden, John D. "The Confederate Retreat from Gettysburg." In *Battles and Leaders of the Civil War,* vol. 3, pp. 420–29. New York: Thomas Yoseloff, 1956.

General Lee assigned Imboden's cavalry brigade the task of guiding the Confederate wounded from the battle of Gettysburg back to Virginia. All the wounded who wanted to leave were loaded in every available wagon, many requisitioned from the surrounding countryside. The wagons were assembled "in one confused and apparently inextricable mass" all along the road from Gettysburg to Cashtown. Late on the 4th of July, a heavy rainstorm began; "the very windows of heaven seemed to have opened." The wounded in the wagons were drenched; the rain and thunder maddened the horses and mules; the noise of thunder and moaning drowned out all attempts to communicate orders; and the retreat began. "Scarcely one in a hundred had received adequate surgical aid," Imboden estimated. The unsprung wagons bounced along the muddy and rutted roads, torturing their passengers. Colonel Imboden frequently heard men beg to be killed. The commander would not allow any wagons to stop, but continued the retreat throughout the night. "Many of the wounded in the wagons had been without food for 36 hours," writes Imboden. "Their torn and bloody clothing, matted and hardened, was rasping the tender, inflamed, and still oozing wounds." Imboden summarizes the experience: "During this one night I realized more of the horrors of war than I had in all the two preceding years."

Irwin, Bernard J. D. "The Apache Pass Fight." *Military Surgeon* 73 (1933): 197–203.

This essay is taken from an official report written in February 1861 by the assistant surgeon of the 7th United States Infantry. Lieutenant Bascom and sixty men were ordered by the commanding officer of the 7th, Colonel Pitcairn Morrison, to go to Apache Pass looking for Chirichua Apaches who had stolen army mules, horses, and cattle. At the pass, he was attacked by several hundred Apaches under their famous war chief, Cochise. Bascom took refuge in the fortified mail station; one man escaped to Fort Buchanan. From there, a rider was sent to Fort Breckenridge for reinforcements while a small detachment was sent to Apache Pass to notify Bascom that help was on the way. This detachment consisted of fourteen infantry soldiers riding mules, one civilian (a recently discharged soldier who had been awaiting transportation home), and the only officer to volunteer, Dr. B. J. D. Irwin.

Irwin led the band on a two-day, 100-mile trek through a blinding snowstorm. Nearing the pass, they attacked a party of Indians guarding cattle; they drove the cattle into the fortified mail station with three Apache prisoners. The cavalry arrived the next day, and Cochise left. Six Indians were hanged when it was discovered that the Indians had killed six men (three civilians from the mail station and three unidentified). Irwin overcame Lieutenant Bascom's resistance to accomplish what he calls the "extreme mode of reprisal." Irwin was awarded the Medal of Honor; this was, chronologically, the first such medal awarded.

Irwin, Charles K. "Visit to the Hospitals on the Field of Chancellorsville, Va." *American Medical Times* 8 (1864): 210–11.

Irwin was surgeon of the 72nd New York and was designated brigade surgeon of the Excelsior Brigade (made up of the 70th, 71st, 72nd, 73rd, and 74th New York). In his military record (in the National Archives) his name is spelled Irwine. In this report, Irwin tells how he crossed the Rappahannock on 10 May with permission of the rebels in order to render assistance to Federal soldiers who had been wounded at the Battle of the Wilderness, fought 5 to 7 May. He brought with him eight wagons loaded with blankets, dressings, medicine, and food; they were ferried over by the Confederates. The Federal medical authorities with the 11th Corps had established a hospital in a large house near Wilderness Church. This hospital was commanded by Surgeon Hewett of the 119th New York, who rapidly distributed the blankets and food to the suffering wounded. The supplies available to Surgeon Hewett and the other ten to twelve captured doctors had rapidly been exhausted, especially since the enemy surgeons had "appropriated nearly all the dressings, chloroform, instruments, hospital knapsacks, etc., which our surgeons had saved." With Drs. Hewett and Asch, Irwin formed an operating staff and performed a number of amputations. Several of the operations were canceled because the wounded soldiers were so ill that they had "no other prospect than speedy relief by death." Irwin states that gangrene was more pronounced at this location than he had ever seen before and attributed this to the poor nutrition of the wounded.

J

James, Westwood Wallace. "This is War—Glorious War: The Diary of Corporal Westwood James." Edited by Michael Musick. *Civil War Times Illustrated* 17 (October 1978): 34–42.

Westwood James arrived at Charlottesville, Virginia, on 26 July 1861. He was a civilian doctor from Alabama, who volunteered to help at the Charlottesville hospitals. He estimated that 1,200 sick and wounded Confederates and 25 wounded Yankees were located in all the buildings of the University of Virginia. More wounded from the Battle of Manassas kept coming in; "every train brings some of our men who have not had their wounds dressed yet, stinking and full of maggots." He was shaken by what he saw in the hospitals: "to see men once strong and spirited brought almost to death's door by disease contracted by exposure in camp." James later enlisted in an Alabama regiment. He became an assistant surgeon, but none of his military medical experiences are covered in this diary. According to the list of doctors of the Army of Tennessee (*Southern Society Historical Papers* 22 [1894]), James passed his army examining board on 9 December 1862 and served as an assistant surgeon with the Sharpshooters, 4th Brigade, Cleburne's Division until he was court-martialed on 31 January 1864. He was murdered in 1868.

Janney, John Jay. "Talking with the President: Four Interviews with Abraham Lincoln." *Civil War Times Illustrated* 26 (September 1987): 33–36.

This article reproduces a memoir written by a Republican politician from Columbus, Ohio, who was present when petitioners were allowed to present their problems to President Lincoln in his office in the White House. An unnamed woman asked for a pardon for her son, who had been sentenced to death for smuggling contraband of war. Janney quotes Lincoln as saying that he cannot overrule the court that had convicted her son of "giving aid and comfort to the rebels by furnishing them with quinine, percussion caps, and other such things which they can't make and must have." The son was executed for smuggling quinine.

Jarvis, Edward. "Sanitary Condition of the Army." *Atlantic Monthly* 10 (October 1862): 463–97.

After a statistical evaluation of the health of the United States Army from 1800 to 1860 and the health of the Army of the Potomac, he concludes that "our Union army is one of the healthiest on record," although the rate of sickness is three to five times that of a group of civilians of the same age. The key to disease prevention, he states, is to prevent crowding. He calculates the amount of space needed in sleeping quarters to prevent the air from becoming fouled.

Jewett, Charles C. "Report from the 16th Regiment Mass. Vols." *Boston Medical and Surgical Journal* 69 (1863–64): 100–3.

The author was detailed as surgeon-in-charge, field hospital of the 2nd Division, 3rd Corps at the Battle of Gettysburg. The new system, in full operation since the Battle of Fredericksburg, places an officer to supervise (Jewett), a medical officer to direct supplies, another to direct records and burials, and three operating surgeons with three assistants appointed by surgical skill without reference to actual military rank. The remaining physicians accompany the troops to supervise evacuation or man field stations to dress the wounds initially. The initial field hospital was "under the brow of Round-top Mountain," too close to the battle. The bursting of shells and the whizzing of minie balls afflicted additional wounds upon the helpless soldiers, "besides disturbing the nervous equilibrium so necessary for the best services of the surgeons." The hospital had to be evacuated in the middle of the battle. The author's corps suffered most of its wounds on the second day, filling the hospital with 1,500 wounded. The author attributes the high surgical mortality to the exhaustion of the men prior to the battle. The author notes that many of the men who had minor wounds returned to the battle before their names were taken by the recorder, so that the official statistics underrepresent the true number of wounded. The Sanitary Commission supplied more medicine and food to the hospital than the regular purveying department. The only individual mentioned by Jewett was Miss Helen Gilson of Chelsea, who had served in the Corps hospital for the previous eighteen months. She cheered the wounded by cheerful conversation, by attending to their wants, and by singing.

Jewett, Charles C. "After-treatment of Amputations and Resections in the Third Corps Field Hospital after Gettysburg." *Boston Medical and Surgical Journal* 70 (1864): 211–16.

Jewett was surgeon of the 16th Massachusetts, acting as primary surgeon at division and corps hospitals. This report includes operations, mortality, and complications at the 3rd Corps hospital after the Battle of Gettysburg.

Johnson, Charles B. *Muskets and Medicine; or Army Life in the Sixties.* Philadelphia: F. A. Davis, 1917, 276 p.

The author was hospital steward for the 130th Illinois. He suffered a severe and prolonged bout with diarrhea when his unit was in Louisiana. He provides many interesting observations about treatment and convalescence. His medical comments are especially important because, after the War, but before he wrote this memoir, Johnson was trained as a physician.

Johnston, David E. *The Story of a Confederate Boy in the Civil War*. Portland, OR: Glass and Prudhomme, 1914, 379 p.

At age sixteen, this lad joined Company D, 7th Virginia. During the War, he kept track of all the original members of the company. This work lists each by name with what became of him.

Killed in battle or died of wounds:	17
Died of disease:	14
Deserted:	12
Discharged (many for medical cause):	29
Transferred to other commands:	6
In prison at end of war:	27
Absent sick at end of war:	8
Surrendered at Appomattox with Lee:	9
Total members of company	122

Jones, Joseph. "Inquiries upon Hospital Gangrene, Addressed to the Medical Officers of the Confederate Army." *Nashville Journal of Medicine and Surgery* 1 (1866): 241–64, 321–32, and 428–34.

Late in 1864, Surgeon General Samuel P. Moore wrote an open letter to Confederate medical officers, asking them to describe their experiences with hospital gangrene. Jones obtained several of the responses and printed them here, without any of his own comments. P. A. Anderson of Ocmulgee Hospital, Macon, presented seven patients, some with autopsy material. He concluded that the disease is not contagious, but is transmitted by direct contact. Jackson C. Chambliss of Winder Hospital, Division 2, Richmond, extracted material that was exuded from an gangrenous wound and injected it into healthy dogs to see if they would develop some sort of disease, thereby proving contagion. The dogs remained healthy. Deering J. Roberts observed that after the Battle of Lovejoy's Station near Atlanta, about 200 rebel wounded were left on the field. They were taken to a building that had never before been used as a hospital. When he saw them about two days later, several had hospital gangrene; he thought the appearance of the disease in new buildings disproved the contagion hypothesis. Other comments

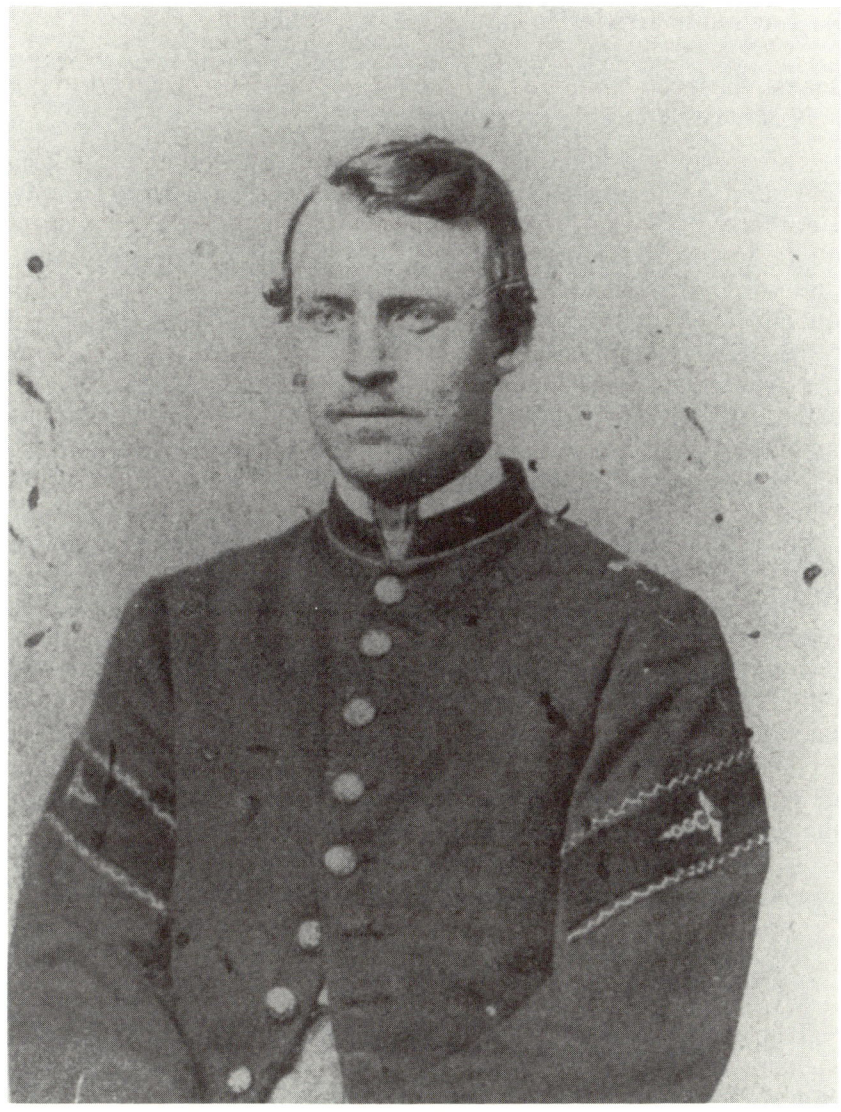

This wartime photograph shows Charles B. Johnson in the uniform of a Union army hospital steward. Johnson carried with him a book on military surgery by the British medical officer Thomas Longmore. From Charles B. Johnson, *Muskets and Medicine*, 1917, opposite p. 128.

were made by Hunter Holmes McGuire, S. C. Merillat, and James A. Fremon of Erwin Hospital, Opelika, Alabama.

Jones, Joseph. *Quinine as a Prophylactic against Malarial Fever.* Nashville, TN: University Medical Press, 1867, 34 p.

This essay is a rambling discussion of many studies of malaria and quinine. He begins by quoting the mortality in Liberty County, Georgia, in the era before quinine was available. He goes on to quote how various English explorers and military leaders used quinine in Africa. He then relates that, during the Civil War, he frequently took quinine personally; on some occasions, he awoke refreshed after taking quinine as he went to bed feverish. During the War, quinine in Confederate forces "failed to yield the most satisfactory result from its irregular and unsystematic employment." Soldiers would not take powdered quinine, but would take it mixed with whiskey. "As a general rule soldiers will not refuse whiskey even when it contains Quinine," he concludes.

To prove the value of the drug in preventing malaria, he instructed Dr. J. N. Warren, assistant surgeon of the 25th South Carolina, in April 1863, to select 200 men of the regiment, then stationed on James Island, and force them to take four grains of quininc per day. Only four of these men developed malaria and only one typhoid fever. The rest of the regiment, some 300 to 400 men, did not take quinine daily; they experienced over 300 cases of malaria and 23 cases of typhoid with 2 deaths. The difference in the incidence of typhoid fever is unexplained; perhaps soldiers debilitated by malaria were unable to obtain clean water.

Jones, Joseph. *Researches upon Spurious Vaccination; or, The Abnormal Phenomena Accompanying and Following Vaccination in the Confederate Army during the Recent American Civil War, 1861–1865.* Nashville, TN: University Medical Press, 1867, 132 p.

This work reviews the problem of inflammation at the site of vaccination. The history of this problem is described in detail. In Jones's opinion, inflammation after vaccination seriously decreased the combat readiness of various military units, especially in the Army of Northern Virginia in the early spring of 1863. Jones concludes that the inflammation was produced by various agents contaminating vaccination material; one outbreak was traced to a prostitute who probably had syphilis. A contributory factor was the generalized debility of the troops, exacerbated by a poor diet.

Jones, Joseph. *Medical and Surgical Memoirs: Containing Investigations on the Geographical Distribution, Causes, Nature, Rela-*

tions and Treatment of Various Diseases 1855–1890, 3 volumes. New Orleans: Clark and Hofeline, 1876–90.

This huge, rambling, discursive work contains most of the same material in the pamphlets above plus a wide variety of other undigested observations and studies. He thinks that the Federal quarantine restrictions kept New Orleans free of yellow fever during the War. Quarantine was opposed by "powerful railroad and steamship interests" and fell into disuse after the War, leading to the terrible epidemic of 1878.

Jones, Joseph. "The Medical History of the Confederate States Army and Navy." *Southern Historical Society Papers* 20 (1892): 109–66.

This article is not a narrative history, but rather a gathering of diverse material. Included are a list of all doctors from the State of Florida who had served in the Confederate States Army, a calculation of the losses in some battles such as Shiloh and Chickamauga, and a list of some of the physicians who were with the Confederate forces inside the fortress of Vicksburg. Jones attempts to estimate the total number of Confederate doctors. The Confederate States Army contained a total of 834 surgeons and 1,668 assistant surgeons, he thinks, while the Confederate States Navy contained 22 surgeons, 10 assistant surgeons, and 41 passed assistant surgeons. Jones discusses the insignia of the Confederate Medical Corps.

Jones, Joseph. "Roster of the Medical Officers of the Army of Tennessee." *Southern Historical Society Papers* 22 (1894): 165–280.

This article lists the medical officers of the Army of Tennessee and its hospital support system. Included is the officer's full name, date of commission, when he passed the army medical boards, and his assignments. The original volume from which this list is taken, now in the Joseph Jones papers at Tulane University, also contains the dates that each officer was on leave.

K

Kean, Robert Garlick Hill. *Inside the Confederate Government: The Diary of Robert Garlick Hill Kean.* Edited by Edward Younger. New York: Oxford University Press, 1957, 241 p.

Kean, head of the Bureau of War, made many medical comments.

He wrote, on 17 May 1863, that Beauregard expected Union operations off the South Carolina coast to be halted by the fever season. He occasionally talked with Surgeon General Moore. On 2 August 1863, Moore expressed outrage at the treatment of Confederate prisoners at Fort Delaware.

Keen, William W. "Surgical Reminiscences of the Civil War." *Transactions of the College of Physicians of Philadelphia* 27 (1905): 95–114. Reprint in his *Addresses and Other Papers,* pp. 420–41. Philadelphia: W. B. Saunders, 1905.

Keen was still a medical student when his teacher, John H. Brinton, who was now a brigade surgeon with the United States Volunteers, prevailed upon him to be assistant surgeon with a regiment of Massachusetts militia. The doctor initially assigned (referred to by Keen as Dr. Smith) had resigned. When Keen complained that he knew very little about medicine and surgery, Brinton replied: "It is perfectly true that you know very little, but, on the other hand, you know a good deal more than Smith." During First Bull Run, Keen received no orders, either from his regimental commander or from superiors in the Medical Service (the regimental surgeon, Keen's immediate superior, had disappeared). Keen tried to make himself useful at a small regimental hospital near the fighting, then moved to Sedley Springs Church where a major hospital was formed. He finally accompanied a wounded colonel to Washington, thus making his escape.

After graduation from the University of Pennsylvania in March 1862, he rejoined the army. He was placed in charge of hospitals in two adjoining churches in Washington; carpenters worked all night to lay boards across pews. Keen was also present at Second Bull Run, in charge of a medical supply train. When the supplies were captured by Confederates, the rebel surgeon became wide-eyed and wreathed in smiles at the incredible bounty. He remained behind in Centreville with the seriously wounded for three days; his only help came from volunteers from the Christian and United States sanitary commissions. He later served in Philadelphia hospitals with Silas Weir Mitchell.

By comparing surgery in his own day with Civil War surgery, he gives a graphic picture of the earlier surgical techniques: infections were so common that some degree of postoperative fever was considered normal and pus laudable; joint injuries always produced severe infection; abdominal wounds were frequently fatal because no one tried to repair a damaged intestine; arterial hemorrhage was often fatal because the hemostatic forceps had not yet been invented; no retractors were used to widen a surgical field. Thermometers were occasionally seen, but seldom used; the surgeon judged fever by laying his hand on the patient's skin. Occasional successes made medical life bearable. He describes the severe head wound suffered by Private Robert Dray Murray, leaving him deaf in one ear and blind in one eye, but then relates how, after the War, Murray became a physician with successes in academic medicine and in the United States Navy.

Keen, William W., Silas Weir Mitchell, and George R. Morehouse. "On Malingering, Especially in Regard to Simulation of Diseases of the Nervous System." *American Journal of Medical Sciences* 48 (1864): 367–94.

The authors discuss the possible simulation of diseases of the nervous system. They had extensive experience with these disorders at the Turner's Lane Hospital in Philadelphia. They are absolutely draconian in their approach; e.g., sneaking up behind a soldier who claims deafness and firing a pistol near his ear, observing to see if he flinches. Another technique is to anesthetize the potential simulator with ether and then to examine him as he is coming out of it, still too groggy to remember what his physical deficits were supposed to be. Another important technique was close observation at unusual times. A soldier with a paralyzed arm is walking into town when a sudden guest of wind blows his cape over his head; before he can stop himself, he has used both arms to catch the cape. Another soldier is mute; a passerby speaks a common greeting and the malingerer, unconsciously, replies. The patient recovered himself, however, and grasped Keen to exclaim: "Thank God, Doctor, you have restored my voice!" The authors never try to differentiate between conscious or unconscious motivation; they assume any dysfunction not caused by bodily damage is purposely feigned in order to escape further exposure to shot and shell.

Kellogg, Florence Shaw. *Mother Bickerdyke as I Knew Her.* Chicago: Unity Publishing Co., 1907, 176 p.

The author met Mrs. Bickerdyke in 1891 and knew her for the last ten years of her life. The portion of the book on her wartime career is mainly taken from other published works, although this work includes a few of Mother Bickerdyke's wartime letters to her children back in Galesburg, Illinois. The book emphasizes Mrs. Bickerdyke's postwar career. She attended the 1898 reunion of the veterans of the Army of the Tennessee. She stimulated Kansas Union veterans to vote for women's suffrage in that state. Her monument in Galesburg quotes General Sherman: "She Outranks me."

Kerr, W. J. W. "Pellagra and Hookworm at Andersonville." *Confederate Veteran* 18 (1910), 69.

The author was the Confederate surgeon-in-charge at Andersonville prison. He states that of the sixty-three Confederate doctors who were at the hospital in 1864, he may be the last one living. His knowledge of disease gained since the War makes him believe that both hookworm and pellagra were "rife" among the prisoners. He found pathological changes in the internal organs typical of pellagra when he performed, with Joseph Jones, 128 autopsies upon deceased prisoners. The disease was not known in the country at that time, but the basic food of the prisoners was cornbread. "The symptoms of pellagra as known now," he concludes, "are identically those of a large number of cases that occurred at Andersonville."

King, John H. *Three Hundred Days in Yankee Prison; Reminiscences of War Life, Captivity, Imprisonment at Camp Chase.* Atlanta, GA: J. P. Daves, 1904. Reprint. Kennesaw, GA: Continental Book Co., 1959, 114 p.

King was a private who served in the 1862 invasion of Kentucky and who was later captured when Vicksburg surrendered. After his release from Vicksburg, he returned home to Georgia. After a few months, he rejoined the Confederate army. While retreating near Sevierville, Tennessee, in January 1864, he was struck in the lower face by a minie ball. The ball fractured his lower jaw and passed through his neck, knocking him from his horse, unconscious. He describes the subsequent harrowing events with great emotion and eloquence. A Union surgeon examined his wound but refused to even try to stop the bleeding, thinking that King would soon die. He stopped the bleeding himself by pressure on the neck. Later he was taken to the Union prison camp near Columbus, Ohio. He describes the horrors of prison life, including a smallpox epidemic. After the war, King became a physician.

King, William S. "Necessity of Maintaining the Physical Strength of Recruits and Soldiers." *American Medical Times* 8 (1864): 191–92.

The author was medical director of the Department of the Susquehanna during the 1863 Confederate incursion into Pennsylvania. Fresh troops from several states were rushed to Harrisburg. So many became immediately ill that King had to establish five general hospitals in that location. When Lee retreated after Gettysburg, this force moved from Harrisburg to Hagerstown, toward Winchester, Virginia (along the present route of interstate highway 81). So many soldiers became sick or exhausted by the march that King had to establish hospitals along the route: at Carlisle, Chambersburg, Waynesboro, and Hagerstown. There were virtually no deaths, but the great loss of manpower virtually crippled this force. King attributes the sickness to the "suddenness of the change of habits and food." The troops should have been "seasoned to their work by a little previous training."

L

Lamb, Robert Scott. "Recollections of Some Old Army Officers."
Military Surgeon 62 (1928): 77–83.

The author enlisted as a private in 1861. He states that the doctor of his regiment "had the reputation of being a good surgeon when he was sober." During the first winter of the War, he developed typhoid fever and was taken by a two-wheeled ambulance to Mansion House Hospital in Alexandria; he described the trip as "unendurable." He worked in Alexandria hospitals as a convalescent nurse under Dr. Edwin Bentley. When Dr. Bentley transferred to the Army Medical Museum in 1865, Lamb went with him. This short essay describes the personalities of several other doctors in Alexandria and Washington.

Lane, Alexander G. "The Winder Hospital of Richmond, Va."
Southern Practitioner 26 (1904): 35–41.

The author graduated in medicine from Tulane University in 1858. He was commissioned a surgeon in the Confederate army on 6 June 1861. He served with the 18th Mississippi and was in charge of the Union wounded after the Battle of Ball's Bluff. Those most seriously injured were sent to the General Hospital at Leesburg and received the same rations and care as the Confederate wounded. He proudly reports an amputation performed on a Vermont man from the 17th Massachusetts; the stump healed so well that there were only a few drops of suppuration from each suture.

When Winder Hospital was organized in Richmond in April of 1862, Lane was placed in charge, and he remained so for the remainder of the war. At twenty-seven years of age he commanded 800 hospital attendants and was responsible for the care of up to 5,000 patients. The hospital was organized into six divisions, each with one surgeon and six assistant surgeons and its own dispensary, laundry, and kitchen. The hospital contained baths, a bakery, sixteen acres of gardens tended by convalescents, sixty-nine dairy cows giving three hundred gallons of milk daily, and a separate commissary with two boats to travel up the Kanawha and make purchases from farmers. In the center of the hospital was a huge latrine with two 10,000 gallon water tanks that were discharged into the hollow every other day, carrying the filth from the hospital grounds into the James River. Mrs. Snowden of Charleston brought imported liquors for the patients. "No medical officer was allowed to touch it under penalty of immediate orders to the field."

The six division heads met with Lane each morning except Sunday and inspected one division, selected at random. Continuing education was provided in regular classes, with each division head responsible for one area of knowledge. During the course of the war, thirty-three assistant surgeons from Winder were promoted to surgeon. Between 1 April 1862 and 1 March 1865, the hospital spent $1,220,000 and admitted 76,213 patients, of whom 11,530 were transferred to other hospitals and 3,259 died. Lane is proud of a clipping from the Richmond *Enquirer,* dated 25 September 1862, that reports the mortality of Richmond hospitals varying from a high of 14 percent to the very lowest, Winder at 6 percent. The chief matron of the first division was Miss Emily Mason, daughter of Senator Mason (of Mason and Slidell fame). This hospital is pronounced as "*wine*-der."

Lathrop, D. *The History of the Fifty-Ninth Regiment, Illinois Volunteers.* Indianapolis: Hall and Hutchinson, 1865, 243 p.

Lathrop, the regimental hospital steward, wrote an excellent history of the 59th Illinois. He included a few medical comments. One soldier received a fearful gunshot wound passing through the back into the lung. Air bubbled out of the wound with every exhalation. Doctors paid no attention to the author's suggestion to suture the wound closed, but when the patient was about to die, the doctors left and the author closed the wound with pressure. The soldier could then breathe and he eventually recovered. "Ignorance is bliss," the hospital steward concludes, "but it is not always safe for the patient."

The surgeon of the regiment, Dr. J. D. S. Hazlett (spelled Haslett in the records of the National Archives) received the nickname "Quinine" from the troops for his efforts to force this bitter medicine down their throats. Once after a fatiguing march, he treated all the soldiers to a "snort" of whiskey; the bitter taste revealed that he had laced their reward with quinine. Dr. Hazlett was killed during the Battle of Perryville, shot in the neck while dressing a soldier's wound. Confederates stripped the doctor's body of his hat, boots, gold watch, and surgical instruments.

Lee, George R. "Scene aboard Ship Loaded with Wounded." *Civil War Times Illustrated* 5 (June 1966): 48–49.

Lee was a private with the 11th Illinois Artillery station in Cairo, Illinois. In February 1862, the steamer *War Eagle* brought wounded from the battle at Fort Donelson to Cairo. Lee was assigned as a nurse to accompany the wounded, about half of whom were Confederates, up the Mississippi to hospitals in St. Louis. He describes two deaths.

Leinbach, Julius Augustus. "Regiment Band of the 26th North Carolina." Edited by Donald M. McCorkle. *Civil War History* 4 (1958): 225–36.

Julius Leinbach (1834–1930) was a musician with the band of the 26th North Carolina. During battle, his duty was to care for the wounded. In this extract from his reminiscences, Leinbach describes the suffering of his regiment at Gettysburg as it was cut down in the wheat field on the first day. He gives details of how he and other band members cared for the wounded, how they loaded most of them on wagons for the difficult trip south after the battle, and how Dr. Warren stayed behind with those who were wounded too severely to travel.

Letterman, Jonathan. *Medical Recollections of the Army of the Potomac.* New York: Appleton, 1866, 194 p.

Written immediately after the War, this short book describes Letterman's service as medical director, Army of the Potomac. The first problem Letterman faced was scurvy; to combat this, he utilized meat broth, "cooks being at first employed night and day." Many original orders and reports are quoted, including Letterman's change of command order (23 June 1862), McClellan's order placing ambulances under medical command (2 August 1862), the change from regimental to division hospitals (30 October 1862), and the reorganization of the medical supply system (4 October 1862). The previous regulations supplying a regiment for three months proved "too cumbersome for active operations, instances being frequent when the whole supply had been left on the roadside." Letterman required a standardized medical chest for each regiment and a standardized medical wagon for each brigade. He justified his oversupply of medical support for the Gettysburg campaign with this motto: "Lost supplies can be replenished but lives lost are gone forever" (p. 157). The author allows himself a tirade against medical officers whose major goal is to prescribe a drug or amputate a limb, but who neglect their primary duty, to maintain the health of the army. "Early in January, 1864," he concludes, "I was relieved, at my own request, from the position of Medical Director."

Lewis, John A. "A Sketch of the Life and Service in the Confederate Army of Dr. John A. Lewis of Georgetown, Kentucky." Edited by Hambleton Tapp. *Kentucky Historical Society Register* 75 (1977): 121–40.

Dr. Lewis wrote this sketch of his Confederate service in 1910. Born in Kentucky in 1841, he enlisted in the 2nd Kentucky Cavalry, commanded first by John Hunt Morgan and later by Basil W. Duke. He was a private throughout the war and became a doctor in later life. This sketch contains no medical observations.

Lewis, John B. "Letter from an Army Surgeon in Maryland." *Boston Medical and Surgical Journal* 69 (1863–64): 45–46.

The author was in charge of the army hospital in Cumberland, Maryland. Union troops withdrew on 15 June, 1863, leaving 400 patients in the hospital. He hid all those who could walk in the surrounding woods; when the rebels came through on 17 June, they inspected the hospital, but took no prisoners.

Lewis, John B. "Reminiscences of a Civil War Surgeon, John B. Lewis." Edited by Stanley B. Weld and David A. Soskis. *Journal of the History of Medicine and Allied Sciences* 21 (1966): 47–58.

The author, the same individual who wrote the above contemporary letter, wrote a summary of his Civil War experiences in later life. He was born on Long Island in 1832 and graduated from New York University Medical School in 1853. In 1861, he was appointed surgeon of the 5th Connecticutt. In April of 1862, he was promoted to brigade surgeon in the Army of the Shenandoah and was later medical director of his division. He assisted in the construction of the 3,000 bed pavilion hospital in Cumberland, Maryland, under the direction of Medical Inspector Barnes (later Surgeon General) and Dr. L. H. Steiner of the Sanitary Commission. He states that if serious infections occurred in one of the pavilions, the patients were evacuated and it was destroyed by fire. Lewis was present during the Battle of Antietam; he reports that on 18 September there was total mingling of medical personnel of the North and South. He states that three doctors were killed in the battle: the physicians of the 12th and 20th Massachusetts and Surgeon White, medical director of General Franklin's Corps, who was shot while ascertaining the best location for field hospitals. [National Archives records of the two Massachusetts regiments name the doctors killed in action: Albert A. Kendall and Edward H. R. Revere.]

Lewis, Samuel E. *The Treatment of Prisoners-of-War, 1861–1865*. Richmond: William Ellis Jones, 1910, 16 p.

Lewis, an assistant surgeon with the Confederate States Army, argues in this pamphlet that the mortality among Union prisoners in Confederate hands was less than among Confederates in Union prisons. The main point of contention is the total number of Union prisoners. The tone of the pamphlet is strident defensiveness.

Lidell, John A. "On Epidemic Cerebro-Spinal Meningitis, or Spotted Fever, with Cases." *American Journal of the Medical Sciences* 49 (1965): 17–29.

The author was an army doctor at Stanton General Hospital, Washington, during 1864, when he encountered a new and "formidable" disease. Three patients developed a high, continuous fever followed by purple spots all over the body, rapidly progressing to death. The cases occurred in patients already hospitalized for other reasons and in widely separated wards; the author could not determine how the disorder spread from one patient to another. One case occurred in a hospital guard. Autopsies showed congested vessels in the brain and effusion over the surface of the cerebral hemispheres. The author reviewed the literature but could come to no conclusion on the nature of the disease. Others had theorized about the value of quinine in treatment, but one of these patients was already taking high doses of that medication to treat malaria at the time he developed this disorder. The reviewer concludes that these patients suffered from meningococcal meningitis.

Lidell, John A. *On the Wounds of Blood Vessels; On the Secondary Traumatic Lesions of Bone; on Pyemia*. New York: Hurd and Houghton, 1870, 585 p., 10 color plates.

These three works, bound together, were commissioned by Frank H. Hamilton as part of his *Surgical Memoirs of the War of the Rebellion*. Very little of this review is based upon the author's own observations. After the Battle of Ball's Bluff (21 October 1861), the author saw many tourniquets improperly applied so that venous bleeding was promoted in wounds without arterial bleeding. As the war progressed, Liddel became convinced that many soldiers who were killed in action actually bled to death on the battlefield. On 25 March 1865, he examined forty-three dead bodies on the field immediately after the battle at Fort Stedman. The cause of death was a head wound in twenty-three, a thoracic wound in fifteen, and an abdominal wound in five. Most of the soldiers shot in the thorax, and all five shot in the abdomen showed a "blanched and exsanguinated appearance." Examination of the clothes and surrounding ground showed that some of them had bled externally and some had bled internally.

Linn, John B. "A Tourist at Gettysburg." *Civil War Times Illustrated* 29 (Sept/Oct 1990): 26.

A Union officer home on leave visited the Gettysburg Battlefield from 6 through 11 July. His manuscript, published here for the first time, contains descriptions of hospitals and medical treatment. The Third Division Hospital in the Catholic Church contained wounded soldiers lying next to each other on boards stretched across the pews; the doctor in charge was a brute, swearing and smoking while "paying no attention to the frequent appeals made to him." A civilian surgeon who was present ministered to one raving soldier and discovered that maggots were already in his unattended wound.

Lister, Joseph. "On a New Method of Treating Compound Fracture, Abcess, etc., with Observations on the Conditions of Suppuration." *Lancet* 1 (1867): 357–59.

This is the first description of Lister's use of carbolic acid to prevent infection in wounds. In retrospect, this is considered the classic breakthrough in the development of antiseptic surgery and is often listed as one of the most important papers in the history of medicine. Readers familiar with the struggle of Civil War doctors against gangrene, erysipelas, and other disorders spreading from one patient to another will see this paper against a background of the growth and dissemination of ideas about disinfectants.

Livermore, Mary A. *My Story of the War: A Woman's Narrative of Four Years Personal Experience as a Nurse in the Union Army.* Hartford, CT: A. D. Worthington, 1887. Reprint. Williamstown, MA: Corner House, 1978, 700 p.

Livermore was an important official with the United States Sanitary Commission. She was present at the Battle of Corinth when a Confederate shell hit her hospital. This book includes the personal stories of several other women, including Mother Bickerdyke. She later wrote a second work that includes a few additional anecdotes: *The Story of My Life* (Hartford, CT: A. D. Worthington, 1899, 730 pages).

Locke, E. W. *Three Years in Camp and Hospital.* Boston: G. D. Russell and Company, 1870, 408 p.

The author, a minister, was not in the army, but was a frequent visitor to army camps and hospitals. He repeated the grim jokes told by patients in the hospitals. He relates, for example, that amputees said that "there is no great loss without some gain; my shoemaker's bill will not be so large as it has been"; or, "Sam Talbott and I are going to buy our gloves together." One must understand something of medical practice to understand the riddle: "Why is our surgeon like our chaplain? Because his is such a *feeling* man."

Logan, Mary. *Reminiscences of the Civil War and Reconstruction.* Carbondale: Southern Illinois University Press, 1970, 324 p.

The wife of General John A. Logan, congressman from southern Illinois, visited Union hospitals at various times. She describes how her husband and others wounded at Fort Donelson were cared for in private homes in the area. Her most poignant moment occurred when a secondary hemorrhage produced sudden death in a wounded soldier who had apparently recovered completely. This work is taken from Logan's book, published by Scribner's in 1913, entitled *Reminiscences of a Soldier's Wife.*

Logan, Samuel. "Prophylactic Effects of Quinine." *Confederate States Medical and Surgical Journal* 1 (1864): 81–83.

The regimental surgeons of eight separate Confederate units gathered statistics for soldiers who refused quinine, for those who took some quinine, and for those who, it was thought, took the bitter medicine daily. Among 230 soldiers who took no quinine, 134 developed fever; of 246 who took some of the medication, 96 experienced fever; of 506 who took quinine regularly, 98 had fever. No effort was made to differentiate malaria from other forms of fever. "It would seem from these statistics," concludes the author, "that, though not an absolute prophylactic, the degree of protective power possessed by the agent fully warrants its use."

Longmore, Thomas. *A Treatise on Gunshot Wounds.* Philadelphia: J. B. Lippincott, 1862, 132 p.

This book, written by a British authority on military surgery, was published in England, but reprinted in the United States by Lippincott. A large number were purchased by the United States Army and distributed. The University of Illinois Library has the copy that belonged to hospital steward Charles B. Johnson; the words "U.S. Army Hospital Department" are stamped upon the cover.

Lyle, William W. *Lights and Shadows of Army Life; or, Pen Pictures from the Battlefield, the Camp, and the Hospital.* Cincinnati: R. W. Carroll and Co., 1865, 403 p.

The author was chaplain with the 11th Ohio. Lyle joined the regiment in 1862 and was assigned hospital duty. He spent much of his time ministering to the dying. Lyle was with the regiment when it was engaged at Second Manassas, South Mountain, and Antietam. Later it was transferred to the western theater and participated in the battles of Chickamauga and Missionary Ridge. Lyle left the army when the regiment ended its three-year enlistment in June of 1864. He includes an appendix, listing every death in the regiment; many died from disease, not a few from accidents.

Lyman, George H. "Some Aspects of the Medical Service in the Armies of the United States during the War of the Rebellion." *Military Historical Society of Massachusetts Papers* 13 (1913): 175–228.

After a general introduction to military medical problems, Dr. Lyman relates his own experiences during the War. He was medical director of a division during the Peninsula campaign; he comments favorably on the introduction of the Letterman system. He was with General William Nelson as he bled to death after being shot by another Union general. Lyman also describes treating the wounded after the Battle of Stone's River.

Lyon, A. A. "Malingerers." *Southern Practitioner* 26 (1904): 558–62.

As a young medical graduate, Lyon was immediate assistant or intern to Felix Formento at the Louisiana Hospital, Richmond. They evaluated a patient named Parsons who looked healthy except that he spoke in a whisper. After much heroic therapy for "aphonia," the doctors gave up and gave him a medical discharge. The next day, Lyon saw him in the Richmond streets, loudly auctioning off his personal goods before returning as a civilian to Louisiana. Formento was still embarrassed by this misdiagnosis when Lyon saw him in 1881. A second case of malingering occurred later when Lyon was surgeon with the 48th Mississippi. In early 1863 near Winchester, Virginia, a soldier named Guess suffered terrible epileptic fits. Lyon observes that all his fits occurred just as he was about to go to picket duty. Lyon cured a seizure by throwing ice water on his wriggling body; Guess jumped up and shouted. The next day, however, he deserted, going to a place "where bullets ceased to fly and fits need never come."

Mc, Mac

McDonald, Cornelia Peake. *A Diary with Reminiscences of the War and Refugee Life in the Shenandoah Valley, 1860–1865.* Nashville, TN: Cullom and Chertner, 1935, 540 p.

Nursing was not for everyone. While a refugee in Lexington, Virginia, Cornelia McDonald offered her services as a nurse. Immediately upon entering the local military general hospital, she was repulsed and nauseated by a patient with a horrible facial wound. As she hurried out of the ward, "my dress brushed against a pile of amputated limbs heaped up near the door." She never tried nursing again.

McGarity, Abner. "Letters of a Confederate Surgeon: Dr. Abner McGarity, 1862–1865." Edited by Edmund Cody Burnett. *Georgia Historical Quarterly* 29 (1945): 76–114, 159–90, and 222–53; 30 (1946): 35–70.

Appointed assistant surgeon, Confederate States Army, on 10 March 1863, Dr. McGarity served first with the 21st Georgia, D. H. Hill's Division, Jackson's Corps, and later with the 61st Alabama during the Battle of Winchester and the valley campaign of 1864. These letters contain little medical information.

McGuire, Hunter Holmes. "Observations Upon the History of Hospital Gangrene in the Army of General T. J. Jackson (Stonewall)." *Nashville Journal of Medicine and Surgery* 1 (1866): 432–34.

In response to a letter asking about hospital gangrene from Joseph Jones, McGuire takes the opportunity of recording several observations. He first saw gangrene in January 1862 during the Romney campaign. Hospitals were especially crowded, and McGuire states that he "attributed the hospital gangrene, and the unhealthy appearance of the wounds generally, to the effect of a foul and impure air, whose vitality had been lowered or depressed by cold." The best way to prevent gangrene was to use tents for hospitals. He saw no gangrene during the Shenadoah Valley campaigns of 1862 (Jackson) or 1864 (Early). If a camp or tent hospital became unhealthy, "the whole encampment was moved to a new and clean piece of ground." After Second Manassas, the troops suffered from severe diarrhea, a diarrhea so watery that "if caught in the hand, it would scarcely have soiled it." He attributed this diarrhea to the consumption of green corn. Hospital wagons did not arrive until two days after the battle and the wounded on the field suffered terribly. "Pyemia carried off hundreds."

McGuire, Hunter Holmes. "Progress of Medicine in the South." *Southern Historical Society Papers* 17 (1889): 1–12.

His recollections of the Civil War emphasize improvisation; he tells how he raised a depressed skull fracture using a table fork with a bent central prong.

McGuire, Hunter Holmes, and George L. Christian. *The Confederate Cause and Conduct in the War Between the States.* Richmond: L. H. Jenkins, 1907, 229 p.

The authors defend the South on many questions including causes of the War and treatment of prisoners. The book contains McGuire's description of the death of Stonewall Jackson, originally published in the *Richmond Medical Journal.*

McIntyre, Benjamin F. *Federals on the Frontier: The Diary of Benjamin F. McIntyre, 1862–1864.* Edited by Nannie M. Tilley. Austin: University of Texas Press, 1963, 429 p.

An enlisted man in the 19th Iowa, McIntyre spent the War years in the Trans-Mississippi theater. He makes many straightforward observations about diarrhea, smallpox, scurvy, and measles.

McKay, Charlotte E. *Stories of Hospital and Camp.* Philadelphia: Claxton, Remsen, and Haffelfinger, 1876. Freeport, NY: Books for Libraries Press, 1971, 230 p.

Mrs. McKay had no special training in nursing but went to Baltimore when she heard about soldiers wounded in the rioting at the start of the War. When the local army surgeon in Frederick, Maryland, notified friends in Baltimore that he needed nurses for his hospital, she volunteered. She was at Frederick when Lee's army passed through on its Maryland incursion that ended at Antietam. She was in Washington when she heard of the Battle of Gettysburg and immediately headed for that town. At Camp Letterman, her main duty was to find and distribute food to the wounded. During Grant's Virginia campaign, she nursed at City Point and at the 5th Corps Hospital.

Macleod, George H. B. *Notes on the Surgery of the War in the Crimea.* Philadelphia: J. B. Lippincott, 1862, 403 p.

The chief surgeon of the British forces in the Crimea, Macleod described the experiences of that War. The sole anesthetic used was chloroform. The mortality of penetrating wounds of the head was 100 percent. Mortality following amputation varied by site:

Arm	22.9% of those operated died.
Shoulder joint	27.2%
Lower leg	30.3%
Knee joint	50.0%
Thigh, lower third	50.0%
Thigh, middle third	55.3%
Thigh, upper third	86.8%
Hip joint	100.0%

Despit this high mortality, Macleod advocated amputation when in doubt; more lives were lost by waiting, he thought, then limbs lost by operating early. This work was reissued in Philadelphia in 1862 because of its relevance to United States surgery.

M

Manigault, Arthur Middleton. *A Carolinian Goes to War: The Civil War Narrative of Arthur Middleton Manigault, Brigadier General.* Edited by R. Lockwood Tower. Columbia: University of South Carolina Press, 1983, 344 p.

The author was commanding officer of the 10th South Carolina and later of a brigade. He had long service with the Army of Tennessee up to the fall of Atlanta. He includes an extensive description of the illness in Corinth, Mississippi, as the Federal army approached that city after the Battle of Shiloh. He felt that the severity and extent of sickness was exacerbated by inadequate medical care.

Mason, Emily V. "Memories of a Hospital Matron." *Atlantic Monthly* 90 (1902): 305–18, 475–85.

The author, from Fairfax County, Virginia, had great trouble making her way south at the start of the War. She served as chief of the Georgia division of the Camp Winder Hospital in Richmond. Her comments about her hospital activities are restricted to anecdotes, predominately concerning how she tried to maintain morale. She gives a terrifying description of the Richmond fire of the early morning hours of 3 April 1865. "Between us and the city lay the penitentiary in flames, and from out of the building poured a hideous throng, laden with booty, and adding to the general uproar by their shouts." The first Federal troops that she saw were a regiment of negro cavalry, who waved their sabers to "our negroes" and shouted: "We have come to set you free!" She later served as a matron in a Federal hospital in Richmond.

Mathers, Augustus Henry. "The Civil War Letters of Henry Mathers, Assistant Surgeon, Fourth Florida Regiment, C.S.A." *Florida Historical Quarterly* 36 (1957): 94–124.

The author graduated with a Doctor of Pharmacy degree from Augusta Medical College in Georgia in 1858. At the start of the War, he ran a drug store in Micanopy, Florida. He wrote many letters to his family during 1861 and 1862 while he served as a surgeon with the 4th Florida. He wrote from Cedar Key, Florida, in November of 1861 that "the chills have quit me for a while at least." In December, his regiment was in Fernadina suffering from measles and mumps. He noted that opium was in short supply; he told family members, who were running his drug store, to increase prices of laudanum and paregoric: "sell them high." By February 1862, his regiment had 150 cases of measles, mumps, pneumonia, and catarrh. Fernadina was evacuated because of a threatened Union invasion, and all his sick were transferred to the hospital at Lake City, Florida.

May, H. C. "Case of Gunshot Injury of the Head." *American Medical Times* 8 (1864): 185–86.

William Sheridan, private of the 1st Missouri Artillery, age thirty-four, was wounded on 19 May 1863 at the siege of Vicksburg. A shell exploded over his artillery piece, killing three and wounding two. When Sheridan awoke, he found himself covered with blood, flowing freely from a scalp wound. He walked two miles to the hospital where the surgeons determined that a round ball had entered his brain through the left parietal bone. Its partially flattened surface could be tapped with a long probe. He was taken to Van Buren Hospital on the west side of the Mississippi; an operation was performed under anesthesia, but the ball could not be removed. After nine weeks at Van Buren Hospital (apparently on a moored steamer), he returned to duty but was bothered by headache. He was discharged on 3 September 1863. Four months later, while in Nashville working as a riverboat laborer, he experienced a minor (unrelated) fever and was admitted to Hospital No. 1. May's examination disclosed a well-healed scalp wound, growing hair, but a sunken area over a round hole that was about one and one-quarter inches in diameter. The wound was so regular that it appeared to have been made by a punch and hammer. The patient recovered from the fever and returned to work. May concludes that this case vindicates conservative surgery or "let well enough alone."

Mayer, Nathan. "A Connecticut Surgeon in the Civil War: The Reminiscences of Dr. Nathan Mayer." Edited by Stanley B.

Weld. *Journal of the History of Medicine and Allied Sciences* 19 (1964): 272–86.

Born in Bavaria in 1838, the author graduated from Cincinnati Medical College in 1857 and began extensive further medical studies in Europe. In early 1861, both Northern and Southern United States medical students studying in Paris argued between and even during classes. Mayer returned to the United States and, upon arriving in Hartford, volunteered as assistant surgeon of the 11th Connecticut. He was sent to New Bern, North Carolina, where his regiment was located. He was placed in charge of thirty patients with typhoid and was gratified that only two died. He was also in charge of the smallpox "hospital," which was a tent in the woods where smallpox victims were cared for by blacks who had supposedly survived a previous attack of that disease. Mayer was the only person who traveled back and forth between New Bern and the tent in the woods. His biggest problems at sick call were malaria, dysentery, and malingering. When a picket was shot in the arm, he went to the site where the wound occurred. He amputated the arm, but found that he had not left enough skin and flesh to close over the end of the bone. He sent the victim to Washington, where more bone was removed and the flap could be sutured shut over the shortened end. Mayer was captured at the Battle of Fredericksburg and taken to Libby Prison in Richmond.

Medical and Surgical Reporter. Volumes 6–13, 1861–65.

This medical journal was published weekly in Philadelphia. The journal fell behind in its schedule so that the date of appearance was several weeks behind the printed date; in 1864, the journal reverted to printing the actual date, leaving a hiatus. In 1865 and 1866, the journal published a series of biographical articles on living New York physicians and surgeons; the author, Samuel W. Francis, obtained much of the information by interview, so this is an important source for biographical data about several leading physicians of the era.

"Military Hospitals at Fortress Monroe." *Harper's New Monthly Magazine* 29 (Aug 1864): 306–22.

The author describes two hospitals within Fortress Monroe: the Chesapeake Hospital, located in a four-story building that was originally a school for young ladies, and the Hampton hospital, built on the pavilion system. The later was opened in August of 1862, and, from then until 26 April 1864, there had been 6,540 admissions with 216 deaths, 1,049 invalided, and 4,491 returned to duty (with 784 remaining). But in the next few days, General Grant sent in his sick and wounded, and the number of patients in the hospital swelled to over 2,000. Many drawings are in the article, including the dog Sport, who "instinctively came to the hospital" when his master was killed and he was wounded. He was treated by the doctor in charge, Dr. Ely M'Clellan, even though he lacked proper papers.

Miller, John G. "Application of Iodine for Arresting the Spread of Hospital Gangrene." *American Journal of the Medical Sciences* 62 (1871): 573.

This one-page report summarizes experience with "a great many cases of hospital gangrene" during the Atlanta campaign. The author was the surgeon of the 11th Iowa, placed in charge of the 17th Corps field hospital. Because the rail line to the north was cut, he was unable to obtain bromine; he applied iodine to the wounds two or three times per day with good results.

Mitchell, John K. *Remote Consequences of Injuries and Nerves, and Their Treatment.* Philadelphia: Lea Brothers, 1895, 245 p.

This book is a follow-up report, after a passage of two or three decades, concerning soldiers who had suffered nerve injuries in the Civil War and had been studied by the author's father, Silas Weir Mitchell. The problem of burning pain, causalgia, is still best treated by hypodermic injections of morphine. The author does not say how often the morphine must be given, but he does claim that pain relief is better if the drug is injected directly into the painful area. A large number of surgical therapies, such as cutting the proximal end of the painful nerve, are now available that were not even considered in the 1860s.

Mitchell, Silas Weir. "The Case of George Dedlow." *Atlantic Monthly* 18 (July 1866): 1–11.

Although this story is fictional, many elements are taken from Mitchell's interviews with wounded Union soldiers. The fictional Dr. Dedlow was the assistant surgeon of the 10th Indiana Infantry Regiment. His horrible story involved the stepwise amputation of all four limbs.

Mitchell, Silas Weir. "Some Personal Recollections of the Civil War." *Transactions of the College of Physicians of Philadelphia* 27 (1905): 87–94.

Mitchell praises Surgeon General Hammond for recognizing that the Medical Service of the United States Army "demanded com-

THE

ATLANTIC MONTHLY.

A Magazine of Literature, Science, Art, and Politics.

VOL. XVIII. — JULY, 1866. — NO. CV.

THE CASE OF GEORGE DEDLOW.

THE following notes of my own case have been declined on various pretexts by every medical journal to which I have offered them. There was, perhaps, some reason in this, because many of the medical facts which they record are not altogether new, and because the psychical deductions to which they have led me are not in themselves of medical interest. I ought to add, that a good deal of what is here related is not of any scientific value whatsoever ; but as one or two people on whose judgment I rely have advised me to print my narrative with all the personal details, rather than in the dry shape in which, as a psychological statement, I shall publish it elsewhere, I have yielded to their views. I suspect, however, that the very character of my record will, in the eyes of some of my readers, tend to lessen the value of the meta-

and 1860 attended lectures at the Jefferson Medical College in Philadelphia. My second course should have been in the following year, but the outbreak of the Rebellion so crippled my father's means that I was forced to abandon my intention. The demand for army surgeons at this time became very great ; and although not a graduate, I found no difficulty in getting the place of Assistant-Surgeon to the Tenth Indiana Volunteers. In the subsequent Western campaigns this organization suffered so severely, that, before the term of its service was over, it was merged in the Twenty-First Indiana Volunteers ; and I, as an extra surgeon, ranked by the medical officers of the latter regiment, was transferred to the Fifteenth Indiana Cavalry. Like many physicians, I had contracted a strong taste for army life and disliking cavalry service, sought plete revision." He notes Hammond's defects, "an impulsive temperament and great self-confidence," that led him into his greatest error, removing calomel from the list of army medications. During the War, Mitchell remained a civilian but served as a contract surgeon in Philadelphia. His novel, *In War Time,* describes his service at the hospital established in the old armory building at 16th and Filbert, where he first became interested in nerve injuries. He arranged for patients with dysfunction of the nervous system to be transferred to his ward (in exchange for a patient of his with some other condition). When this ward overflowed with such patients, Hammond arrange for a separate building, Moyamensing Hall on Christian Street. This hospital opened on 5 May 1862 and closed on 29 October 1864. Here he worked with George Morehouse and William W. Keen; Dr. I. P. Reese of the regular army was the surgeon-in-charge. [Actually, many of these recollections are in error.]

When this building in its turn overflowed, a suburban estate was obtained on Turner's Lane; one ward was assigned to Dr. J. M. Da Costa to study heart disease while the remainder was for patients with nervous diseases. Surgeon Alden was in charge and took care of all the military "red tape business." [The administrative physicians, Reese and Alden, were never heard of again while Da Costa, Mitchell, Morehouse, and Keen performed major research and developed important postwar careers.] Mitchell states that at this hospital, atropine was injected hypodermically to control muscle spasms. So many patients with excruciating nerve pain were in the hospital, that, in one year, 40,000 injections of morphine were used. Mitchell reports he has never encoutnered such nerve lesions in civilian practice.

Mitchell, Silas Weir. "The Medical Department in the Civil War." *Journal of the American Medical Association* 62 (1914): 1445–50.

Mitchell's last article, appearing after his death, describes his own experiences in detail, first at the hospital in the Armory at 16th and Filbert, later at the Hospital for Nervous Diseases at Turner's Lane. The great mass of disorders of the nervous system was unprecedented. "The opportunity was indeed unique, and we knew it." He took over 1,000 pages of notes. He blames Morehouse for losing notes on exhaustion (neurasthenia) in a fire. Mitchel describes hospital gangrene and informs his audience, "you will never see it." He relates Hammond's accomplishments, but then adds that Hammond suffered "defects of character which were increased by the applause which greeted the success of his radical measures." He summarizes the medical experiences of the Civil War with this phrase: "We had served faithfully as great a cause as earth has known."

Mitchell, Silas Weir, George R. Morehouse, and William W. Keen. *Gunshot Wounds and Other Injuries of Nerves*. Philadelphia: J. B. Lippincott, 1864. Reprint, with an introduction by Ira M. Rutkow. San Francisco: Norman Publishing, 1989, 164 p.

This detailed study of gunshot wounds of nerves includes detailed case reports, giving the soldier's units, geographic location when wounded, exact position when wounded, passage of the ball, immediate symptoms, symptoms when transferred to Turner's Lane Hospital for Nervous Disorders, Philadelphia, treatment, and subsequent course. The work contains the first description in man of damage to the cervical sympathetic nerve, later called Horner's syndrome, and the first description of the burning nerve pain later called causalgia (and still later, reflex sympathetic dystrophy).

Mitchell, Silas Weir, William W. Keen, and George R. Morehouse. "On the Antagonism of Atropia and Morphia, Founded upon Observations and Experiments Made at the U.S.A. Hospital for Injuries and Diseases of the Nervous System." *American Journal of the Medical Sciences* 50 (1865): 67–76.

After a lengthy introduction describing how experimentation with human beings gives superior results to animal experimentation, the authors relate their observations upon soldiers with pain due to gunshot injuries involving peripheral nerves. This pain was relieved only by subcutaneous injections of morphine. Pain relief was superior if the morphine was injected near the painful nerve. The experimenters also gave atropine by subcutaneous injections to these same injured soldiers. Atropine caused no pain relief. If atropine was given with morphine, the two drugs had some antagonistic effects. Morphine alone constricted the pupil, while atropine alone dilated the pupil; together they caused less change in pupillary size (but the effect of the atropine lasted longer). Morphine caused drowsiness, but atropine caused visual illusions; together these two effects tended to cancel each other. Atropine did not change the pain relief produced by morphine, nor did morphine change the sensation of dry mouth caused by atropine. This is a basic study of human pharmacology; the practical result suggests that atropine can lessen the bothersome drowsiness produced by morphine without changing pain relief.

Monteiro, Aristides. *War Reminiscences by the Surgeon of*

Mosby's Command. Richmond: C. N. Williams, 1890. Reprint. Gaithersburg, MD: Butternut Press, n.d., 236 p.

This memoir covers Monteiro's experiences with Mosby in northern Virginia during the last year of the War. The author, a medical graduate of the University of Virginia, provides mainly military descriptions. Perhaps the greatest medical interest is Monteiro's relationships with Yankee surgeons.

Moore, J. P. "Gun-shot Wound of the Head." *Southern Practitioner* 26 (1904): 551–53.

The author joined the Confederate States Army early in 1863, just in time to be surrendered at Vicksburg. He was assigned to the 10th Tennessee (with every member but one an Irishman) immediately prior to the Battle of Chickamauga. Of the 157 men of the regiment present at that battle, 100 were killed or wounded. In the field hospital the day after the battle, he came across a prewar friend, Colonel J. L. McCullum. His hair and clothes were matted with dried blood. He had been shot in the center of the forehead with the ball passing through the center of the brain and exiting the top of the skull. Moore carefully cut his hair, cleaned his body and head, cut off the brain tissue that protruded from both wounds, tightly bandaged the head, and evacuated him to the general hospital system. After the War, Moore and McCullum both lived in Yazoo City, Mississippi. McCullum ran the newspaper and did not suffer from "the slightest loss of mental vigor or muscular power."

Moore, Samuel P., ed. *A Manual of Military Surgery Prepared for the Use of the Confederate States Army, Illustrated.* Richmond, VA: Ayres and Wade, 1863. Reprint. San Francisco: Norman Publishing, 1989, 297 p.

This book is full of exact detail and graphic drawings showing precisely how to perform an operation. An inexperienced medical officer might use this book to perform an amputation that he had never previously performed—or even seen. The manual was prepared by a committee. The members were not mentioned in the body of the work, but included Jesse J. Abernethy and Alexander N. Talley, who was president of the Richmond Board of Medical Examiners.

Moore, Samuel P. "Indigenous Remedies of the South." *Confederate States Medical and Surgical Journal* 1 (1864): 106–08.

The Surgeon General of the Confederate States Army surveys the medicinal properties of plants. "A bountiful Providence has spread over the broad surface of our Southern land all the elements of an independent nationality," he boasts. But then he complains that the American Medical Association has failed to ask the United States government to allow medicines to pass the blockade. "This learned and powerful tribunal of the medical profession of the North" has become "forgetful of the noble and unselfish teachings of the healing art—blind to all save the gratification of a ruinous hate and ungratified revenge."

Moore, Samuel P. "Grand Summary of the Sick and Wounded of the Confederate States Army under Treatment during the Years 1861 and 1862." *Confederate States Medical and Surgical Journal* 1 (1864): 139–40.

This brief editorial summarizes the statistics of sickness and death available to the Surgeon General's office for the first two years of the War. The original returns were lost in the Richmond fire and this is the only source of this information.

Morrow, Maude E. *Recollections of the Civil War from a Child's Point of View.* Lockland, OH: John C. Morrow, 1901, 48 p.

The author was only eight years old in 1862 when she and her mother traveled to Corinth to attend to her severely ill father, Coridon Morrow, who was assistant surgeon of the 43rd Ohio.

Morton, William T. G. "The First Use of Ether as an Anesthetic at the Battle of the Wilderness in the Civil War." *Journal of the American Medical Association* 42 (1904): 1068–73.

This article was taken from a manuscript made during the War by Dr. Morton, credited as the discoverer of anesthesia. The title is misleading since both ether and chloroform were used extensively throughout the War to produce anesthesia. Morton went to the Virginia battlefields in 1864 to, as he puts it, "administer the pain-destroying agent which it pleased God to make me the human agent to introduce for the benefit of suffering humanity." Of course, many others were administering anesthesia on both sides of the battle line. Nevertheless, Morton's report is jammed with interesting observations.

As he headed for the battlefield, he encountered the walking wounded. "It is the most sickening sight of the war, this tide of wounded flowing back. One has a shattered arm, and the sling in which he carries it is the same bloody rag the surgeon gave him the day of battle; another has his head seamed and bandaged so you can scarcely see it, and he weaves like a drunken man as he drags along through the hot sun; another has his shoe cut off, and a great roll of rags wound around his foot, and he leans heavily on a rough cane broken from a pine tree; another breathes painfully and holds his hand to his side, where you see a ragged rent in his blouse; another sits by a puddle, dipping water on a wounded leg, which, for want of dressing since the battles, has become badly inflamed; another lies on a plot of grass by the roadside, with his browned face turned full to the sun, and he sleeps. So I passed hundreds in riding a few miles." At field hospitals, he administered anesthesia for many operations. He was impressed by the dexterity of the surgeons and, especially, the rapidity of the operations. "Scores" were completed in the same time that one would be performed in peacetime.

Moses, Israel. "Surgical Notes of Cases of Gunshot Injuries Occurring during the Advance of the Army of the Cumberland in the Summer of 1863." *American Journal of the Medical Sciences* 47 (1964): 324–42.

Moses was medical director of the Army of the Cumberland. He describes the Federal hospitals in Murfreesboro and the treatment of the Confederate wounded who remained behind after the Battle of Stone's River. The report contains medical statistics and many case reports of individual wounded soldiers.

Moses, Israel. "Surgical Notes of Cases of Gunshot Injuries Occurring near Chattanooga, Tenn., in the Battles of Sept., Oct., and Nov., 1863." *American Journal of the Medical Sciences* 48 (1864): 344–66.

The author was medical director of the Chattanooga complex of hospitals from the time it was evacuated by the rebels on 9 September until he was relieved of duty on 15 November 1863. The retreating Confederates had stripped the city of medical supplies, but left several good hospital buildings. Moses increased the hospital capacity of the city to 3,000 beds. The city filled to "every nook and corner" after the horrible battle of 19 and 20 September—the battle that was "a disaster to our arms" (he cannot even write the word Chickamauga). He estimates that two of every nine soldiers in the army were killed or wounded in that battle. The rebels captured a great deal of medical supplies including ambulances. The Union wounded poured into the city by every imaginable form of transportation. The author rails against the policy of moving each wounded soldier to his correct division hospital. He also opposed the utilization of civilian physicians, who came from the North to help, but who had too little surgical experience to be of much aid.

Murray, William D. "The Alarms of the Peninsula Campaign: A

Letter of Surgeon Murray of the 100th Regiment." *Niagara Frontier* 15 (1960): 57–60.

Murray was assistant surgeon of the 100th New York. In a letter dated 14 July 1862, he describes the widespread feelings of despair after his regiment was chewed up at Fair Oaks on 31 May.

They were forced to retreat, leaving the dead and wounded on the field. The surgeon of the regiment, Martin S. Kittenger, together with the hospital steward, Frank Cook, stayed behind with a group of wounded and were taken prisoner. During the retreat on the Peninsula, Murray noted that the company commander, Captain Lewis S. Payne, was delirious with fever. On his own iniative, he relieved him of command, kept him quiet throughout the night, and the next day led him to the rear on Kittenger's horse.

N

Neil, Alexander. "The Leg that Broke Loose: Recollections of the Battle of New Market." Edited by Richard R. Duncan. *Civil War Times Illustrated* 19 (January 1981): 43–45.

Neil was assistant surgeon with the 12th West Virginia. He describes the Battle of New Market in a letter to his family. Neil assisted removal of Federal wounded to a small church, where he dressed wounds until informed that the Union forces were retreating; he ordered the removal of the wounded, but rode off before many had been evacuated. The title does not refer to a human leg, but to a metaphor for the Union strategy for 1864 (one army will hold a leg of the Confederate bear, while other armies skin it).

Newberry, John S. *The U.S. Sanitary Commission in the Valley of the Mississippi During the War of the Rebellion, 1861–1866.* Cleveland: Franklin, Benedict and Company, 1871, 543 p.

This work is full of statistics, official reports, and firsthand observations. In September 1861, the Western (or St. Louis) Sanitary Commission declined Newberry's offer of a merger and determined to take care of the region west of the Mississippi River, while the Western Division of the United States Sanitary Commission provided support to military activities in Tennessee. Newberry narrates Sanitary Commission activities after the battles of Fort Donelson, Shiloh, Murfreesboro, Chickamauga, and Chattanooga as well as during the Vicksburg, Atlanta, and Nashville-Franklin campaigns.

Newton, Edwin M. "Reminiscences of the Medical Department,

Confederate States Army and Field and Hospital Service, Army of Northern Virginia." *Southern Practitioner* 26 (1904): 168–74.

Newton includes a letter from Francis Sorrell, written in 1902, who states that when he arrived in Richmond from California to join the staff of the Surgeon General's Office on 15 August 1861, he saw medical chaos much worse than anything he had seen during seven years of medical service with the United States Army. All the sick from the new troops plus the wounded from First Manassas filled Richmond. Sorrell was put in charge of general hospitals; worse was to come. After the Seven Days battles, Richmond's population of 40,000 was swelled by 20,000 patients in hospitals. Newton goes on to list other important medical officers in Richmond and in the Army of Northern Virginia. Medical directors of Corps were: 1st (Longstreet's) J. S. Cullen; 2nd (Jackson's) Hunter McGuire; 3rd (A. P. Hill's) J. W. Powell, who died in Mississippi of yellow fever during the epidemic of 1878; Cavalry Corps J. B. Fontaine, who was killed while attending a wounded officer, General Donovan.

Newton served at Hospital No. 1, directed by Charles Bell Gibson. Also serving at the hospital was St. George Peachy, who had been in the Crimean War with the British at Scutari. Dr. E. J. Ethridge, who had served with the Russians at Sevastopol, was senior surgeon with Cobb's brigade. Newton describes the nursing services at Hospital No. 1: Catholic nuns from Baltimore under the direction of Sister Valentine. He mentions many other doctors, such as Jones Berrien of Georgia, who had been in the United States Army. He was with the Army of Northern Virginia, serving directly under Hood and later was medical purveyor for the Trans-Mississippi Department. J. C. Herndon, also previously with the United States Army, died of yellow fever while serving with Confederate forces at Fernandina, Florida. Joseph E. Claggett of Maryland was in charge of the Receiving and Forwarding Hospital and of transporting all sick and wounded from the Army of Northern Virginia to Richmond.

Nightingale, Florence. *Notes on Hospitals.* London: Longman Green, 1858, 187 p.

Nightingale wrote this short book about hospital construction after she had visited most of the hospitals of Europe, as well as the best and the worst hospitals for British forces in the Crimea. The British hospital at Scutari, Turkey, was built in a former Turkish army barracks. The sewer system under the building had rotted away, and, it was discovered later, the hospital water system flowed through the decaying body of a dead horse. Needless to say, the hospital mortality was frightful; over 40 percent of the patients admitted died. This could be compared to another British hospital near the Turkish village of Renkioi, which had been built out of small, temporary buildings with good control of a clean water supply and a sewage disposal system. Of the 1,331 admissions to Renkioi, only 50 patients died.

Nightingale described the ideal hospital as a series of separate oblong buildings with cross ventilation. She felt that the key to a healthful hospital was ventilation to carry away the vapors from the skin and lungs of the sick, "the exhalations from whom are always highly morbid and dangerous." The worst sort of construction was exemplified by the recently completed Royal Victoria Hospital, where the effluvia from one patient must pass across all the others in a row before escaping out a window. These separate buildings or wards in the ideal Nightingale hospital had water closets all at one end, where the waste was washed away, and were connected at the other end to a corridor that connected to other wards, to doctor's and nurse's quarters, and to the kitchens. This book was extremely influential and went through several editions in Britain and in the United States.

Nightingale, Florence. *Notes on Nursing: What It Is, and What It Is Not.* London: Harrison, 1859, 79 p.

This simple and popular book is based upon the thesis that all women are basically nurses. "Every woman, or at least almost every woman, in England has, at one time or another of her life, charge of the personal health of somebody, whether child or invalid,—in other words, every woman is a nurse." The book then gives some straightforward practical advice on how to be a better nurse. The nurse, for example, should not leave the patient's untasted food by his side in the hopes that he might take a bit of it sometime. This leads to a general disgust of food. "Let the food come at the right time and be taken away at the right time, eaten or uneaten." This was an immensely popular work in England and in the United States, going through many editions and reprinted many times.

Nightingale, Florence. *Directions for Cooking by Troops in Camp and Hospital.* Richmond: J. W. Randolph and Co., 1861, 35 p.

Florence Nightingale sent a report to the United States War Department on healthful cooking. Most of the material was taken from her previously published *Notes on Nursing.* Although the Union War Department did nothing with this material, a copy was somehow obtained by Confederate Surgeon General Samuel P. Moore, who ordered it printed for the use of the Confederate army.

O

O'Keefe, D.C. "Surgical Cases of Interest, Treated at Institute Hospital, Atlanta, Ga., May and June, 1864." *Confederate States Medical and Surgical Journal* 2 (1865): 25–33.

The surgeon-in-charge of the Institute Hospital in Macon, Georgia, presented the details of fifty-four soldiers experiencing gunshot wounds during the first two months of the Georgia campaign. Most patients were transferred from the battlefield, through Atlanta, to Macon in only one or two days.

Olmsted, Frederick Law. *Hospital Transports: A Memoir of the Embarkation of the Sick and Wounded from the Peninsula of Virginia in the Summer of 1862.* Boston: Ticknor and Fields, 1863, 167 p.

This work contains descriptions, by Olmsted and others, of problems treating and evacuating the sick and wounded from the Peninsula by boat. The major problem was a conflict of authority. According to Olmsted, the boats belonged to the government which retained authority; the Sanitary Commission had reconstructed the interior of the vessels and, therefore, only had authority of events occurring within the boats. So who could order these vessels to move? Olmsted had a major argument with the medical director of the Army of the Potomac; he states that he always followed the director's orders but he was very disappointed in his lack of organization. The director, unnamed, was Charles Tripler, whose negative opinion of the Sanitary Commission is given in his official report in the *Official Records,* series 1, vol. 11, pp. 196–203.

Olmsted, Frederick Law. *The Papers of Frederick Law Olmsted: Vol IV, Defending the Union: The Civil War and the U.S. Sanitary Commission, 1861–1863.* Edited by Jane Turner Censer. Baltimore, MD: John Hopkins University Press, 1986, 757 p.

These collected letters are important to understand the organization of the United States Sanitary Commission and the efforts of private individuals to reform the United States Army Medical Bureau. Olmsted was present during the Peninsula campaign and frequently quarreled with Charles Tripler, the medical director of the Army of the Potomac. Olmsted called Secretary of War Stanton "the meanest kind of small, cunning, short sighted, selfish politician" (p. 399), and is it is not surprising that Stanton fought with William Hammond, the surgeon general who owed his position to Olmsted.

Ordronaux, John. *Hints on the Preservation of Health in Armies.* New York: D. Appleton and Co., 1861. Reprint. With an introduction of Ira M. Rutkow. San Francisco: Norman, 1990, 142 p.

This brief survey of military hygiene is especially interesting because it was completed in May 1861—before the start of hostilities. The main stimulus for the work was the British finding that soldiers of their peacetime army were twice as likely to die of disease as civilian men of the same age. Ordonaux bases most of the work on the study of European publications. European measures, such as kilograms, are sometimes used, and European military ideas are frequently expressed, such as different physical qualifications for riflemen and "infantry of the line." There are chapters on marching, on camp cleanliness, on food, and on clothing. A chapter on examination of the recruit was enlarged into another book published two years later. An appendix includes the official report of a U.S. Army Board (consisting of C. A. Finley, C. S. Tripler, and R. H. Coolidge) convened to decide whether the army should rely on two-wheeled or four-wheeled ambulances.

Ordronaux, John. *Manual of Instructions for Military Surgeons on the Examination of Recruits and Discharge of Soldiers.* New York: D. Van Nostrand, 1863. Reprint (bound with above 1861 work by Ordronaux). San Francisco: Norman Publishing, 1990, 234 p.

This work was written at the request of the United States Sanitary Commission to be used by examining physicians to determine if a volunteer or draftee was physically fit to join the United States Army. The author states that the work is based upon similar manuals for the Prussian and French armies. The emphasis is upon differentiating symptoms that are due to true disease from those that are feigned. "Many passages in the manual bear an impress of obscurity," admits the author, "which, it is almost needless to say, has been purposely given them, in order not to furnish any instruments of deception to those who might seek here for assistance in accomplishing themselves in the art of malingering." If a recruit alleges the presence of a disease that is not obvious, the examiner should suspect malingering. "In cases of doubt, it is always safest to assume the disease as feigned, rather than real." The same rules apply to a veteran soldier who hopes to obtain a medical discharge from the army.

Otis, George A. *Reports on the Extent and Nature of the Materials Available for the Preparation of a Medical and Surgical History of the Rebellion.* Philadelphia: J. B. Lippincott, 1865, 166 p.

This work was originally a circular from the Surgeon General's Office. It surveys the material that was available for the construction of the *Medical and Surgical History.* It includes case reports, pictures, and preliminary tables of the results of operations such as amputation.

Otis, George A. *A Report on Amputations at the Hip Joint in Military Surgery.* Washington, DC: Government Printing Office, 1867, 87 p., 9 color plates.

This work consists of detailed descriptions of many soldiers who suffered injury to the upper femur, forcing amputation or disarticulation of the leg at the hip joint. The best results were obtained when the initial operation removed the leg by cutting through the femur at a high level; weeks to months later, a second operation disarticulated the stump.

Otis, George A. *A Report on Excisions of the Head of the Femur for Gunshot Injury.* Washington, DC: Government Printing Office, 1869, 141 p.

This report gives the detailed histories of soldiers who were shot in the upper thigh and underwent removal of the damaged portion of the bone without amputation. Otis is not reporting his personal experience, but is summarizing all operations performed during the War by surgeons North and South.

Otis, George A. *A Report of Surgical Cases Treated in the Army of the United States from 1865 to 1871.* Washington, DC: Government Printing Office, 1871, 296 p.

This work contains brief summaries of many surgical cases treated after the War. It is most notable for the first case of a quadruple amputee; all four of his limbs developed gangrene following severe frostbite.

Owen, Urban G. "Letters of a Confederate Surgeon in the Army of Tennessee to His Wife." Edited by Enoch L. Mitchell. *Tennessee Historical Quarterly* 4 (1945): 341–53; 5 (1946): 60–81, 142–81.

Owen was born in Williamson County, Tennessee, in 1833 and graduated from the Medical Department of the University of Pennsylvania in 1855. After one year as resident at the New York Hospital, Owen entered medical practice in his hometown. At the beginning of the War, he enlisted in the 20th Tennessee as a private, but was later surgeon of the 4th Tennessee. Jones (cf. *Southern Historical Society Papers* 22 [1894]), who spells Owen's first name Urbane, states that Owen was appointed surgeon of the 4th Tennessee on 31 December 1862 even though he did not pass his army examining board (at Shelbyville, Tennessee) until 3 June 1863. After the Battle of Murfreesboro, Owen states that "for three days, the surgeons were all very busy." About three hundred wounded men were "crying doctor, doctor at the same time." He was himself quite ill from fever about three months later; he was "reduced to a skeleton." After the Battle of Chickamauga, the entire battlefield smelled of putrefaction.

P

Packard, John Hooker. *A Manual of Minor Surgery.* Philadelphia: J. B. Lippincott, 1863. Reprint. San Francisco: Norman Publishing, 1990, 288 p.

The author was a young but well-trained Philadelphia surgeon. During the Civil War, he was an acting assistant surgeon in several United States Army hospitals in Philadelphia. He traveled to Gettysburg to perform operations during and following that battle. In 1863, he wrote the present book on minor surgical operations, including many operations for gunshot wounds. An official United States Army committee consisting of J. H. Brinton and J. J. Woodward approved the book. A most interesting chapter is entitled "Disinfectants"; it argues that certain diseases such as dysentery and gangrene travel from patient to patient, carried by infected particles in the air. Packard calls these particles "fomites." Certain chemical preparations including chlorine can counteract this mode of disease transmission. Heat also can stop the transmission, and Packard recommends that bedding and clothing should be heated in a stove or boiled in water between uses. The author's son, Francis Packard, became a noted medical historian.

Page, William H. "Letter." *Boston Medical and Surgical Journal* 66 (1862): 478–81.

This letter to the editor is dated 21 June 1862 from Savage Station, Virginia. The author reports the health of the 3rd and 4th Corps to be good, despite the fact that they were forced to occupy swampy ground. He has begun to see cases of scurvy, however. The report describes several wounded soldiers in detail. Page operated by candlelight all night on May 31st. When he finally went to his room to sleep, he found the entire room filled with wounded. He slept in a small tent but a heavy rain "drenched me both above and below."

Page reports that most Union soldiers were wounded with round balls, very few with the conical minie ball. He assisted a South Carolina surgeon operate on thirty captured rebels. Only one minie ball was recovered; the others had passed directly through the flesh. He thinks that the conical bullet used by Union forces is producing much more fearful wounds than the rebel musket balls. He thinks that the army will push into Richmond soon, and such a mass of wounded as he has encountered "is something not likely to occur again in our time."

Page, William H. "I Shall Be a Prisoner." Edited by Roy Zarruchi and Carolyn Page. *Civil War Times Illustrated* 30 (September 1991): 42.

This memoir was written by Page in 1887. He was a well-known Boston surgeon (a protégé of Oliver Wendell Holmes) when he went to Europe in 1860. He encountered many other physicians, from both the North and the South, who became more feverish in the weeks preceding the fire on Fort Sumter. Most higher class Europeans, thought Page, favored the South because they wanted to see the United States, which they called the "American Bubble," broken up into several smaller European-like nations: "the sooner it bursts the better."

Upon his return to Boston, the governor of Massachusetts appointed him to accompany McClellan's forces on the Peninsula, then to return with the first contingent of the wounded of his state. He operated extensively after the Battle of Fair Oaks; cannon balls hit near the hospital. Later, after the Seven Days battles, McClellan retreated, leaving about 3,000 wounded behind. Dr. Page was one of those who volunteered to stay with the wounded. Unfortunately the retreat was only a few hundred yards, so that the advancing Confederates first shelled the hospital, and then, when told of their error, an artillery battle ensued over the heads of the wounded and their doctors. When the Federals retreated farther, Page and the wounded were ordered by Confederates to march into Richmond. Most of the wounded were unable to walk, so Page influenced the rebels to maintain their captivity at Savage Station. There they remained for six weeks, with many medical and supply difficulties, but were eventually exchanged, leaving City Point on the *Daniel Webster*. It is interesting to compare the account of James Winchell, a wounded soldier who was at Savage Station and was repatriated on the same steamer.

Parker, Francis Lejau. "The Battle of Fort Sumter as Seen from Morris Island." *South Carolina Historical Magazine* 62 April 1961): 65–71.

Dr. Parker was an assistant surgeon in the Confederate States Army. His eyewitness account of the bombardment of Fort Sumter, 11 to 13 April 1861, contains absolutely nothing of direct medical interest.

Parker, William Warren. *Reminiscences of Field Hospital Service with the Army of the Potomac.* Buffalo, NY: Buffalo Medical and Surgical Journal, 1889, 27 p.

William W. Parker was assistant surgeon with the 49th New York during the Peninsula campaign and the Battle of Antietam. He was surgeon with the 57th New York during the Battle of Gettysburg and the Virginia campaign of 1864. [I was unable to read this work.]

Parsons, Emily Elizabeth. *Memoir of Elizabeth Parsons.* Boston: Little, Brown, 1880, 159 p.

Emily Parsons had been unwell almost since her birth in Cambridge, Massachusetts, in 1824. Childhood accidents left her blind in one eye with poor vision in the other eye and hard of hearing, and she walked with a limp. In 1861, at the age of thirty-seven, she lived a retiring life with her family. She shocked her father when she told him that her contribution to the cause of the Union was to become a nurse. Unlike many other men and women, who rushed to war in a romantic surge, Miss Parsons arranged for special nurse training. Her father used his influence to obtain a special position for her at Massachusetts General Hospital.

After one year of training, she volunteered for service at the military general hospital at Fort Schyler, New York. Mrs. Fremont convinced her that her skills were needed in St. Louis, and she became a nurse at Lawson Hospital in that city. She took charge of nursing services on board the steamer *City of Alton,* evacuating the sick and wounded from Vicksburg. She was later made chief of nurses at Benton Barracks Hospital, a huge organization occupying the amphitheater and buildings of the St. Louis Agricultural Society. At its height, the hospital housed 2,500 patients including newly freed slaves. Her father, writing the introduction to this series of letters to her family back in Massachusetts, still has trouble understanding how a shy, retiring, disabled maiden could rise to such an important position. He attributes it to her unremitting fearlessness.

Patten, James C. "An Indiana Doctor Marches with Sherman: The

Diary of James Comfort Patten." Edited by Robert G. Athearn. *Indiana Magazine of History* 49 (1953): 405–22.

Patten graduated from the Ohio Medical College in 1849. He joined the 58th Indiana as assistant surgeon on 12 April 1864. He observed that scurvy was becoming a potentially severe problem in his regiment in July 1864. The surgeon of the regiment, Dr. Samuel E. Holtzman, obtained a keg of pickles from the United States Sanitary Commission and distributed it to the men; although there was only about one-half of a pickle for each man, this helped abort scurvy. Patten was present at the Battle of Jonesboro and marched with Sherman from Atlanta to the sea, but he made few medical comments in his diary. He left military service in Savannah on 31 December 1864 when the 58th Indiana was mustered out.

Peddy, George W. *Saddle Bag and Spinning Wheel; Being the Civil War Letters of George W. Peddy, M.D., and his Wife, Kate Featherstone Peddy*. Edited by George Peddy Cuttino. Macon, GA: Mercer University Press, 1981, 332 p.

Peddy graduated from the New Orleans School of Medicine in 1859 and became the surgeon of the 56th Georgia. He participated in the Kentucky invasion of 1862, the battles of Chickamauga and Chattanooga, the Atlanta campaign, and Hood's invasion of Tennessee. These letters from a regimental doctor to his wife are very touching, but contain virtually nothing on his professional duties.

Pember, Phoebe Yates. *A Southern Woman's Story: Life in Confederate Richmond*. New York: G. W. Carleton, 1879. Reprint. With an introduction by Bell Irvin Wiley. Jackson, TN: McCowat-Mercer Press, 1959; Reprint. St. Simons Island, GA: Mockingbird Books, 1987, 199 p.

A matron from Chimborazo Hospital describes her work in detail. She dressed wounds by herself, cooked special diets in her own kitchen, and fought rats, both the four-legged type and the miscreant convalescents termed "hospital rats." The night Richmond burned, the hospital guards left, and Pember protected the alcohol supply with a loaded pistol in order to prevent the hospital rats from drunken debauchery. She knew the War was lost when she saw the fine uniform and horse of the first Union soldier to enter Richmond. This is one of the great books to come out of the War.

Perry, John Gardner. *Letters from a Surgeon of the Civil War*. Boston: Little, Brown, 1906, 225 p.

John G. Perry was born in Boston in 1840, entered Harvard College in 1858, and was trained at the Scientific School. He attended Boston Medical School but had not yet graduated in 1862 when he became a United States Army contract surgeon, assigned to the hospitals at Fortress Monroe, Virginia, where he assisted a Dr. Cushing. On 3 July 1862, Fortress Monroe received 1,000 wounded from the battles on the Peninsula. Later, he was in charge of the medical care of black workers. Twenty had measles, but their skin was "so confoundedly black" that this Boston Yankee could not see their measles spots. In 1863, he returned to Boston and graduated from Boston Medical School; he was given academic credit for his military medical experience. He became assistant surgeon with the 20th Massachusetts and was with them through the summer campaign in Virginia. His journal ends abruptly on 13 August 1864. He seldom writes about his medical activities, but on one occasion he succinctly describes his surgery: "I am up to my neck in work. It is slaughter, slaughter."

Peters, DeWitt C. "Interesting Cases of Gunshot Wounds." *American Medical Times* 8 (1864): 3–4.

The author, surgeon-in-charge of Jarvis General Hospital, Baltimore, describes four patients wounded at Gettysburg. "Private W. E." of the 5th Massachusetts Artillery was wounded on 2 July by a minie ball traversing from his left abdomen to his right buttock. When examined by Jarvis on 13 July, the abdomen was distended and knees were drawn up in pain. Gas and feces escaped from both wounds and from his urethra when pressure was placed on the abdomen. The case was hopeless, "and so I informed him." With cleaning of the wounds, frequent changes of dressing, injection of tea into the bladder, enemas, opium, and a good diet, the soldier recovered. He returned home on 18 September 1863.

"Sergeant W. R.," age twenty-three, 7th New Jersey, was knocked unconscious on 2 July. When he regained consciousness, he staggered to the field hospital and was told by the doctor that "you cannot possibly live." When examined by Peters on 10 July he found a small hole in the forehead as round as if it had been trephined. He inserted his little finger into the hole as deeply as it would go; the edge of the wound was smooth. He thought that the ball was still back farther in the brain substance. The patient complained of dizziness and headache, but could walk and had "no diminution of muscle power or thought." After frequent dressings, he recovered enough so that he could return home on leave on 12 August. Upon his return fifteen days later, reexamination showed the wound was still open, so the soldier was transferred to the 2nd Battalion of the Invalid Corps.

Peters, Dewitt C. "Gunshot Wound of the Internal Carotid and Vertebral Arteries—Fracture of the Atlas—Secondary Hemorrhage and Death." *American Journal of the Medical Sciences* 49 (1865): 373–74.

A private identified by his initials, I.I., of the 187th New York, age twenty-seven, was shot in the mouth at the battle at Hatcher's Run on 6 February 1865. The musket ball entered his mouth, loosening several upper and lower teeth. The surgeon felt inside the mouth, but was unable to find the ball; the private thought he might have swallowed it. On 11 February, he was admitted to the Jarvis Hospital in Baltimore. He walked about the ward and even requested the medical attendant to remove a loose tooth. The next day, however, at about 5:30 P.M., secondary (late) hemorrhage occurred. Bright red arterial blood gushed from his mouth. The patient fainted from loss of blood. The doctor pressed on both common carotid arteries to try to stop the bleeding. The mouth was forcibly opened and the doctor pressed upon the posterior throat. The bleeding was better controlled with carotid pressure, and eventually it stopped. Dr. Peters considered an exploratory operation to look for the site of bleeding but thought the patient too weak to survive. Ice was kept on the throat throughout the night, but, the next morning, blood again gushed from the mouth, and the patient bled to death. An extensive autopsy was performed. The first cervical vertebra or atlas had been fractured by the ball, which was still in the bone.

Porcher, Francis Peyre. *Resources of the Southern Fields and Forests: Medical, Economical, and Agricultural.* Charleston: Evans and Cogswell, 1863, 601 p.

The author was asked by Surgeon General Moore to survey the flora and fauna of the Confederacy in order to identify local materials that could be used in the War effort. This work is a massive listing of all plants throughout the Southern states with suggestions of their medicinal value. Modern analysis of Porcher's recommendations are mixed, but the present reviewer thinks that this work contains nothing of modern medical importance. The author's name is pronounced "Porshay."

Porcher, Francis Peyre. "Confederate Surgeons." *Southern Historical Society Papers* 17 (1889): 12–21.

The author, who was in charge of major Confederate hospitals in Norfolk and Petersburg, states that he never experienced a severe shortage of supplies, although he used civilian donations to supplement government issues. Nevertheless, he concludes that "we could not expect to compete with the highly-organized and lavishly-supplied medical and surgical departments of the United States of the North."

Potter, David D. *The Naval History of the Civil War.* New York: Sherman Publishing Co., 1886, 843 p.

This interesting history was written by a major Union naval officer. The book covers the river war, the blockade, and the chasing of Confederate raiders. While the work contains no direct discussion of naval medical care, it includes occasional comments on specific medical activities. Assistant surgeon William Longshaw, for example, was killed in action during the final attack on Fort Fisher, North Carolina, while treating wounded sailors from the assault party. Several large tables list all the ships and their officers, including medical officers, in various fleets at various times.

Potter, William W. *Reminiscences of Field Hospital Service with the Army of the Potomac.* Buffalo: Buffalo Medical and Surgical Journal, 1889, 27 p.

This pamphlet is reprinted from the *Buffalo Medical and Surgical Journal.* Potter was assistant surgeon with the 49th New York and participated in the Peninsula campaign. He was promoted to surgeon with the 57th New York in January of 1863. His regiment participated in the battles of Chancellorsville, Gettysburg, the Wilderness, and Spottsylvania. He remained with the regiment until it was mustered out on 2 December 1864.

Powers, Elvira J. *Hospital Pencillings.* Boston: Edward L. Mitchell, 1866, 211 p.

Powers worked as a nurse in several hospitals during the last year of the War. The book is in the form of a diary, but, from its organization and narrative content, it was obviously written later. She worked at Hospital Number 1 in Nashville and at the smallpox hospital in that town (where most of the patients, she thought, had measles, not smallpox). She spent most of her time at Jefferson General Hospital, Jeffersonville, Indiana, located directly across the Ohio River from Louisville, Kentucky. She entered nursing on 1 April 1864 with absolutely no experience.

She described the Jefferson Hospital: twenty-four wards radiating from a circular corridor like spokes from a wheel. Each ward was 22 by 150 feet and contained, at most times, fifty-nine beds. The surgery and kitchens were located within the inner circle. She noted that she could work all day, walking many miles, without ever going outdoors. She gives many interesting observations, such as the time that Federal convalescents were "turned out of warm quarters" to make room for newly arriving wounded Confederates. She noted huge overcrowding following the Battle of Nashville; the overflow were put on mattresses on the floor. A Union soldier wounded at Franklin remained in rebel hands for about three weeks. He reported that four out of the five rebel doctors deserted and of the original 287 wounded prisoners, only 163 were alive when the Federals retook Franklin. This is a valuable description of life in a support hospital in the west during the last year of the War.

Pryer, W. C. "Hospital Gangrene in the DeCamp General Hospital." *American Medical Times* 8 (1864): 4–6

DeCamp General Hospital on David's Island, New York Harbor, was built to handle wounded Confederates. Between 17 and 25 July, the hospital received nearly 3,000 rebels wounded at Gettysburg. The author had eighty of the most seriously wounded in his pavilion, plus less seriously wounded ones in surrounding tents. The great majority of the eighty developed hospital gangrene, but none died. His treatment regimen was: first, clean the alimentary canal with mercury; second, give oral tonics including quinine; third, wash the wound with creosate and other materials (Pryer was unable to obtain bromine). "Each patient was supplied with a sponge for his own use solely" and these were washed daily. The wounded prisoners were encouraged to spend as much time as possible outdoors.

Q

Quintard, Charles Todd. *Doctor Quintard: Chaplain CSA and Second Bishop of Tennessee, Being his Story of the War.* Edited by Arthur Howard Noll. Sewanne, TN: University Press of Sewanee, 1905, 183 p.

Quintard served in the War mainly as a chaplain, but he was also trained as a doctor. On several occasions, he obtained leave from his position as chaplain and volunteered his services as an assistant surgeon. These reminiscences are most notable medically regarding the battles of Chickamauga and Franklin. After Chickamauga, he was sent with 150 ambulances to remove the wounded. The Federal wounded were taken to field hospitals that had been set up and were directed by Union doctors. He described one young boy desolate because the Georgia doctor had told him that his leg must be amputated. Quintard examined the wound and told the boy that the leg could easily be saved. He personally took him to the general hospital and later learned that the doctor "had come up from Georgia to get a little practice" of amputation. After the Battle of Franklin, Quintard carried some wounded soldiers to the residence of John McGavock, "whose house and grounds were literally filled with the Confederate dead and wounded." He gives details of the deaths of the six Confederate generals.

R

Reed, William Howell. *Hospital Life in the Army of the Potomac.* Boston: William V. Spencer, 1866, 199 p.

An agent for the United States Sanitary Commission, Reed was with the hospital support system of the Army of the Potomac. He was at the 9th Corps Hospital after the Battle of Fredericksburg, was at the hospital in White House, Virginia, following the Battle of Cold Harbor, and helped in several hospitals during the siege of Petersburg. Reed describes the transport and treatment of the wounded; many specific individuals are described in detail.

Reyburn, Robert. *Fifty Years in the Practice of Medicine and Surgery, 1856 to 1906.* Washington, DC: Beresford, 1907, 39 p.

Reyburn was born in Glasgow, Scotland, but immigrated to the United States at an early age. He was an assistant surgeon at Mansion House Hospital in Alexandria for several years during the War. In 1865, he was surgeon-in-charge of the Freedman's Hospital. After the War he was chief medical officer of the Freedman's Bureau; he kept the medical record after the shooting of President Garfield and testified in the trial of the assassin Guiteau. [I was unable to read this work.]

"The Richmond Ambulance Corps." *Southern Historical Society Papers* 25 (1897): 113–14.

Several of the citizens of Richmond formed a committee to supply ambulances. The ambulances served at most of the battles of the Army of Northern Virginia, beginning in 1862. They accompanied Lee in the Pennsylvania incursion that ended at Gettysburg. This article lists those citizens who served the ambulance corps.

Rogers, James B. *War Pictures: Experiences and Observations of a Chaplain in the U.S. Army, in the War of the Southern Rebellion.* Chicago: Church and Goodman, 1863, 258 p.

The author was chaplain with the 14th Wisconsin. Despite some hospital experience, he has little to say about medical care, with the exception of a heartrending description of surgery after the Battle of Shiloh. The wounded were brought from Shiloh to the small town of Savannah, Tennessee, by steamer on the Tennessee River. They were unloaded and carried to a double log house that was used as a hospital. "Those only who have seen numbers together for amputation can have any idea of the dreadful scene we witnessed. In the open space between the two houses was the table on which the subjects lay for amputation, while the apartments on either side were full of the wounded, waiting their turn. At one end of this open space, under the stairs, lay a pile of legs and arms which had been severed from the maimed and bleeding trunks." The chaplain thought that the operating surgeon was unnecessarily brutal.

Ropes, Hannah Anderson. *Civil War Nurse: The Diary and Letters of Hannah Ropes.* Edited by John R. Brumgardt. Knoxville: University of Tennessee Press, 1980, 149 p.

The author was a nurse at the Union Hotel Hospital in Washington. She describes her visit to the Surgeon General's Office on 1 November 1862. When the pompous Hammond failed to respond to her complaints about her orderly, she went to the secretary of war, who had the orderly arrested.

Ryan, Andrew *News from Fort Craig, New Mexico, 1863.* Edited by Ernest Marchand. Santa Fe, NM: Stagecoach Press, 1966, 72 p.

The letters from a private with the 1st California contain a few medical comments. The regiment was with the California Column traveling from Fort Yuma to New Mexico. Ryan's company occupied Fort Craig during most of the War years and experienced frequent skirmishes with Apaches. Ryan states that only three soldiers in his regiment died during the War: one from tuberculosis, one killed by the Apaches, and one killed by the accidental discharge of a rifle.

S

Schuppert, Moritz. *A Treatise on Gun-shot Wounds: Written for and Dedicated to the Surgeons of the Confederate States Army.* New Orleans: Bulletin Book and Job, 1861, 47 p.

This pamphlet was published separately after initially appearing in the *New Orleans Medical and Surgical Journal.* It described treatment of various injuries from gunshot wounds, mainly of the limbs. Amputation was de-emphasized. The author, born and trained in Germany and having moved to New Orleans only in the early 1850s, based this work upon previous publications, mainly those of Esmarch and Stromeyer, leading German military surgeons.

Schurz, Carl. *The Reminiscences of Carl Schurz,* 3 vols. New York: McClure, 1907–8.

In his memoirs, General Schurz concentrates on military matters. But, after the Battle of Gettysburg, he toured the division hospital and left a riveting eyewitness account of battle surgery: "As a wounded man was lifted on the table, often shrieking with pain as the attendants handled him, the surgeon quickly examined the wound and resolved upon cutting off the injured limb. Some ether was administered and the body was put in position in a moment. The surgeon snatched the knife from between his teeth, where it had been while his hands were busy, wiped it rapidly once or twice across his blood-stained apron, and the cutting began. The operation accomplished, the surgeon would look around with a deep sigh, and then: 'Next!'"

Sheeran, James B. *Confederate Chaplain: A War Journal of Rev. James B. Sheeran, c.ss.r., 14th Louisiana, C.S.A.* Edited by Joseph T. Durkin, with a preface by Bruce Catton. Milwaukee, WI: Bruce Publishing, 1960, 168 p.

This Catholic chaplain made a few observations about the wounded. He visited the Federal wounded on the field after Second Manassas and found them in a "deplorable condition." Late in the War, he obtained a pass from General Sheridan to visit the Confederate wounded left behind as Sheridan drove up the Shenandoah Valley.

Silliman, Justus M. *A New Canaan Private in the Civil War: Letters of Justus M. Silliman, 17th Connecticut Volunteers.* Edited by Edward Marcus. New Canaan, CT: New Canaan Historical Society, 1984, 117 p.

Silliman, a private with the 17th Connecticut, gives an interesting description of his wounding the first day at Gettysburg. He suffered a blow to the head: "I experienced a curious sensation in the head, on opening my eyes I found myself in a horizontal position and surrounded by Greybacks." With other wounded, he was kept a prisoner in a building in town. He was amazed at his kind treatment; "those who a short time previous had been hurling death at

us, now assisted our wounded, bringing them water, crackers, etc."
The following day, he was taken by ambulance wagon to the German Dutch Reformed church at the edge of town. Union doctors were present in this hospital, but they "were more neglectful to our wounded than were the rebel doctors." They watched the battle from the church windows. He observed a ferocious charge by the famous Louisiana Tigers. When the Confederates retreated, they left the Union wounded. Silliman remained in the hospital at Gettysburg, mainly as a nurse, until late September.

Sims, J. Marion. *The Story of My Life.* New York: D. Appleton, 1884, 471 p.

Sims was the leading gynecological surgeon of his day. This work is his autobiography up to 1863; the remainder of his life is filled out with his letters edited by his son, H. Marion-Sims. Sims was born in South Carolina in 1813 and graduated from Jefferson Medical College in 1835. He was famous for devising a surgical treatment of vesico-vaginal fistula using silver sutures. In the 1850s, he suggested that silver sutures could close wounds of the bowel, preventing their fecal contents from leaking into the abdomen; no such operation was attempted during the Civil War. He spent most of the War in Europe. During the Franco-Prussian War, he organized a volunteer medical unit that served at the siege of Sedan.

Smiley, Thomas T. "The Yellow Fever at Port Royal, S.C." *Boston Medical and Surgical Journal* 67 (1863): 449–68.

An outbreak of yellow fever killed, among others, the commanding general, Ormsby Mitchel (a leading American scientist before the War). Smiley presents a map that shows the progression of the disorder. Individuals affected by yellow fever did not pass the disorder to others such as their medical attendants; therefore, concludes the author, the disease is not contagious.

Smith, Adelaide W. *Reminiscences of an Army Nurse during the Civil War.* New York: Greaves, 1911, 263 p.

The author performed volunteer nursing work in Union hospitals, particularly at City Point during Grant's Virginia campaign. She gives many specific case details. When a severely wounded soldier asked for barley broth, she ransacked all available sources. She finally obtained one package of broth from the Christian Commission, brewed it, and served it with "my special attractive little array of silver cup, dainty doiley, etc." This kind of personalized attention must have done wonders for morale.

Smith, Isaac, Jr. "An Incident in Army Practice." *Boston Medical and Surgical Journal* 71 (1864): 340.

While on duty as assistant surgeon, 26th Massachusetts, the author was called to attend the delivery of a pregnant black woman, a laundress at the Port Hospital, New Iberia, Louisiana. The woman delivered twins, both of whom died. One of the babies was very light-skinned, the other very dark. The white baby possessed features that "would have done honor to an American mother" ("American" meaning white American) while the darker skinned baby had "the true African build." The author argues that his observation proves that twins can be produced by two different fathers. He wrote this article while recuperating at his father's home in Foxboro. He had been shot in the right foot while treating wounded at the Battle of the Opequan near Winchester, Virginia, on 19 September 1864.

Smith, Susan E. D. *The Soldier's Friend.* Edited by John Little. Memphis, TN: Bulletin Publishing Co., 1867, 300 p.

The author first became involved in hospital work while tending to her son, a Confederate soldier. She became a matron at Newsom Hospital, Memphis, named for Ella Newsom. This hospital was moved to Chattanooga after the fall of Memphis, where she remained as matron. She transferred to Ford [actually Foard, named for the medical director of the Army of Tennessee] Hospital in Ringgold, Georgia. She helped to evacuate this hospital to Calhoun, Georgia. She was in the Direction Hospital in Chattanooga, working under a Dr. Lytle, when the Federals began to shell the town. She helped in the emergency evacuation of the hospital supplies and patients to Calhoun, then to Griffin, Georgia. She later served as matron at Hill Hospital, named for A. P. Hill. After the Battle of Missionary Ridge—which she viewed from a great distance— the sick were taken to Empire Hospital in Atlanta, and the hospital supplies and staff were relocated to Covington, Georgia, in the buildings of the former Female Institute. During the battle for Atlanta, Federal troops occupied Covington and took all the hospital attendants prisoner, except for one who played the role of a patient. The patients were not bothered, but the surgeon-in-charge, Dr. William H. Robertson, was taken prisoner briefly. She remained at this location for most of the rest of the war. The last eighty pages of the book consist of letters of appreciative patients and doctors to Mrs. Smith, many of whom call her Mother Smith. Sometimes her patients called her "the old grandma."

Souder, Mrs. Edmund A. [Emily Bliss Thacher]. *Leaves from the*

Battle-field of Gettysburg. Philadelphia: Caxton Press of C. Sherman, 1864, 142 p.

This book consists of letters written to her husband by a woman who went to Gettysburg to offer help after the battle. She arrived on 15 July after some difficult travel and distributed her beef broth to the hungry convalescing wounded. She then served as a volunteer nurse at the 2nd Corps Hospital. She was still present when the national cemetery was dedicated on 19 November. She heard Lincoln deliver his address; to her, he appeared the "chief mourner."

Spencer, Newton B. "The Court-Martial of Private Spencer." *Civil War Times Illustrated* 27 (February 1989): 35–40.

Private Spencer was disgusted at the excessive losses suffered at the Battle of the Crater, fought near Petersburg on 30 July 1864. He wrote a letter to a newspaper critical of military authority. This article contains exerpts from his subsequent court-martial and the offending letter, the latter of which contains some interesting medical observations. Spencer states that his unit, Company F of the 179th New York, left Elmira, New York, in June with eighty men and three officers. As he writes, on 12 August, the company has dissipated in this manner:

Killed in action:	4
Wounded, in hospital:	18
Died of wounds:	4
Missing in action:	2
Sick, in hospital:	22
Deserted:	12 ("tough bounty jumpers")
Detached to artillery:	8
Present for duty:	10

Of the three officers, one accompanied the detachment to the artillery, one is sick in the hospital, and the company commander, Allen T. Farnell, was officially missing but had been wounded when last seen. "God grant that he may still be living," writes Spencer, "and be yet enabled to return in health to his dear ones at home." Unfortunately, the military record of Captain Allen T. Farwell of the 179th New York (in the National Archives) states he was killed in action on 30 July 1864.

Stearns, Amanda A. *The Lady Nurse of Ward E.* New York: Baker and Taylor, 1909, 312 p.

Most of this book consists of Amanda Akin's letters to her sisters. She worked at Armory Square Hospital, Washington, from April of 1863 to July of 1864. The hospital was a newly built structure, located between the Smithsonian Institute and the Capitol, convenient to the steamboat landing. The surgeon-in-charge was Dr. D. Willard Bliss, who was arrested (but later reinstated) when a discharged orderly went directly to Secretary of War Stanton with claims that the doctor was pilfering funds. The daughters and wives of many leading Washingtonians visited the hospital at one time or another. Miss Akin often saw President Lincoln visit the hospital, shaking hands with each soldier and saying, "God bless you."

The author describes the arrival of the wounded from the Battle of Chancellorsville; the first contingent of about 150 were brought in on wagons in the early hours of the morning with the only illumination by lanterns. The next day the hospital was crowded with a maze of visitors, especially the members of local relief societies searching for wounded from their states. On 9 July 1864, the hospital received the sudden order that "every man able to carry a musket" should be ready to leave tomorrow to repel a rebel raid (Jubal Early's). Several patients are referred to by name with details of their conditions; some are only referred to by their bed numbers. One patient, Captain Constantine Lippe, refused leg amputation, but seemed to be improving when Miss Akin left the hospital on 20 July 1864. [Lippe's military record in the National Archives states he was discharged from the army on 4 November 1864.]

Steiner, Lewis Henry. *A Sketch of the History, Plan of Organization, and Operations of the U.S. Sanitary Commission.* Philadelphia: J. B. Rodgers, 1866, 13 p.

The author graduated from the medical faculty of the University of Pennsylvania in 1849. During the War, he was an official with the United States Sanitary Commission. This brief summary of the Commission presents his personal observations on the health of the Army of the Potomac during the Virginia campaign of 1864.

Stevens, George T. *Three Years in the Sixth Corps.* Albany, NY: S. R. Gray, 1866, 436 p. Second edition. New York: Van Nostrand, 1867, 441 p. Revised edition. New York: Van Nostrand, 1870, 449 p.

The author was surgeon with the 77th New York. His regiment had nearly 1,000 healthy soldiers when it arrived on the Peninsula in March of 1862, but only about 250 when it left in August. The author remained with this regiment in the Army of the Potomac, engaged at Antietam, Gettysburg, the Wilderness, Spottsylvania, and Cold Harbor. He left military service when the regiment was mustered out after three years service on 13 December 1864. After the War, Stevens became a pioneer neuro-ophthalmologist. [I was unable to read this work.]

Stevens, George T. *On Excisions in Cases of Gunshot Wounds.* Albany, NY: Van Benthuysen, 1866, 13 p.

This very interesting pamphlet describes the author's personal experience with excision, an operation that removes the damaged portion of a bone but saves the limb. A typical case is Captain George M. Ross of the 77th New York, wounded at the battle of Winchester on 19 September 1864. A minie bullet passed through his right arm near the shoulder, shattering the humerus. The author "excised the injured part of the bone, sawing so high as to include a part of the great tuberosity." His arm was immobilized by bandages and later, at the general hospital, by a plaster of Paris cast. His arm was shortened by about an inch, but retained such good function that he returned to his regiment.

Stevenson, Benjamin Franklin. *Letters from the Army, 1862–1864.* Cincinnatti: W. E. Dibble and Co., 1884, 311 p.

Stevenson, a medical graduate of Transylvania University, was surgeon of the 22nd Kentucky (Union). He wrote frequent informative letters to his wife. He was older than most medical officers in the field, passing his fifty-second birthday while in the army. His regiment served the first year near Cumberland Gap, but then moved to the Mississippi. He operated extensively after the battles of Chickasaw Bluffs and Arkansas Post. The army suffered from widespread sickness. "We are sending daily hundreds of men to the up-the-river hospitals," he wrote on 26 January 1863, "and yet the sick accumulate here faster than we know what to do with them." In the 22nd Kentucky, 71 men had been evacuated to the hospitals in Memphis (most of whom had been wounded), 40 men had deserted, 48 were on the sick list but with the regiment, and 301 men were fit for duty.

He accompanied Grant in his move south of Vicksburg. During the siege of that stronghold, he was in charge of the 9th Division Hospital, located in the house and yard of a retired merchant. The hospital was visited by Medical Inspector Summers, who did not make a good impression. "He is just as much a charlatan professionally," concluded Stevenson when Summers recommended soap dissolved in turpentine to stop the bleeding after an amputation, "as he is a blackguard, braggert, and bully officially." Dr. Madison

Mills, medical director of the 13th Corps, pulled Stevenson aside and told him to remain silent and let the inspector "have full swing." During the siege, Stevenson saw a minie ball pass through three soldiers, killing the first (this occurred among Union soldiers arguing over a card game). After the fall of Vicksburg, Stevenson served in Louisiana until February of 1864, when he resigned.

Stevenson, William G. *Thirteen Months in the Rebel Army.* New York: A. S. Barnes and Burr, 1862. Reprint. New York: A. S. Barnes and Co., 1959, 160 p.

Stevenson was forced to enlist in the rebel army while visiting in Arkansas at the start of the War. He became sick in 1861 while in Bowling Green and was evacuated to Nashville, where he was treated by Dr. Stout. Stevenson witnessed the death of General A. S. Johnston at Shiloh; he thinks that his life could have been saved by a tourniquet. While a convalescent in Corinth, he entered hospital service, considering himself an assistant surgeon under Dr. J. C. Nott. He accompanied sick and wounded soldiers on a harrowing train ride to Mobile and later to Selma.

Stout, Samuel H. "Some Facts of the History of the Organization of the Medical Services of the Confederate Armies and Hospitals." *Southern Practitioner* 22–25 (1900–03).

In a rambling narrative broken into twenty-two articles, each six to eight pages in length, an important leader in the Army of Tennessee gives his reminiscences as he approaches eighty. Stout began the War as the surgeon of the 3rd Tennessee (Confederate). The regiment was scheduled to go to the Virginia theater, but 650 of its soldiers were disabled by measles, six of whom died. Stout attributed this huge outbreak of measles to the excessive use of whiskey. He discusses the shifting medical leadership of the Army of Tennessee as the commanders of the army changed. B. W. Avent was medical director while the army remained under state control. D. W. Yandell became medical director of the western theater while A. S. Johnston held overall command there. When Johnston was killed at Shiloh and Beauregard and then Bragg took control of the Army of Tennessee, A. J. Foard became medical director. E. A. Flewellen became medical director of the Army of Tennessee when Foard accompanied Joseph Johnston to Richmond. Foard returned, however, and was medical director, Army of the Tennessee, under Generals Bragg, Johnston, and Hood. He was exhausted by the war and died of tuberculosis in 1868.

Stout became medical director of the General Hospitals of the Army of Tennessee. He was quite proud of his organization of the hospitals of Chattanooga. When the Confederacy evacuated that town, the hospitals were moved south, maintaining their names, staff, supplies, and patients. These hospitals included the Academy Hospital, named for an academy on a ridge in Chattanooga. Under Frank Hawthorne, the hospital was moved to Atlanta and then to Auburn, Alabama. Gilmer Hospital was built on the pavilion system in Chattanooga, named for Mrs. Gilmer of Pulaski, Tennessee, who aided sick soldiers in Bowling Green. Under Charles E. Michel, the Gilmer moved to Marietta, Georgia and then to Auburn. The Newsome Hospital, also newly built in Chattanooga, was named for Mrs. Ella Newsome, who helped sick troops at Corinth. Under the direction of A. Hunter, the hospital moved to Atlanta and later to Thomaston, Georgia.

Stout said that his greatest problem concerned the quartermasters and the commissaries, who failed to furnish needed materials. He bought from many sources personally, using cotton as a form of money when suppliers would not accept Confederate script. Stout sent medical officers directly to Wilmington and Charleston to purchase supplies that had come through the blockade. He hired his own quartermaster, George E. Fairbanks, later treasurer of the University of the South, and even his own fisherman, Cousin John Thrasher, who went to Florida, caught fish, and returned to supply hospitals. When he could not obtain hospital forms from government sources, Stout obtained a printing press from a Chattanooga newspaper to print his own forms.

Stout's narrative, although rambling, is full of interesting detail. Wounded and sick arriving at Atlanta were examined by doctors at the railway station to see what hospital they should go to. After a major battle, these doctors stood on their feet so long, working so frantically, that their feet swelled and their boots had to be cut off.

Strong, George Templeton. *Diary of George Templeton Strong,* 4 volumes. Edited by Allan Nevins and Milton H. Thomas. New York: Macmillan, 1952.

Strong was the secretary of the United States Sanitary Commission. His very frank diary provides a great deal of information on the Commission and on Hammond's appointment as Surgeon General, United States Army.

Swank, Luther. "Inflation Grips the South: Luther Swank Reports from a Field Hospital." Edited by Horace Mathews. *Civil War Times Illustrated* 22 (March 1983): 44.

This article contains two letters from Luther Swank, hospital steward of the 15th Virginia. One of his duties was to shop for supplies for the brigade hospital (Case's Brigade, Pickett's Division, Army of Northern Virginia). He made his purchases at the 6th Street Market in Richmond and was amazed at how prices shot up throughout 1864. There are no medical observations.

T

Taft, Charles S. "Last Hours of Abraham Lincoln." *Medical and Surgical Reporter* 12 (1865): 452–54.

This report is a medical analysis of the last hours and the autopsy of Lincoln, written by a young army surgeon who was the second doctor to reach the stricken president. When he examined the president in the house across the street from Ford's theater, he found him unable to swallow, with his right pupil widely dilated. The left side of the face twitched and the president pronated both arms upon his chest. After about seven hours, the president's breathing underwent a change, varying from deep and regular to periods of no breathing. Each prolonged apnea produced a "death-like stillness" in the crowded room. Many present would look at their watches to note the time of death, but then respirations would slowly begin again, building to deep movements, then slowing to another period of apnea. At 7:22 A.M. the breathing finally ceased. The autopsy showed that the ball, a homemade derringer bullet, had entered the president's neck just to the left of the midline, crossed the center of the brain, and lodged behind the right eye, fracturing both orbits.

Tarbell, Eli M. "Civil War Medicine: A Patient's Account." Edited by David A. Rausch. *Pennsylvania Folklife* 26 (Summer 1977): 46–48.

Sargeant Eli M. Tarbell of the 19th United States was wounded near Atlanta on 28 May 1864. His diary reveals the problems of his treatment and his evacuation to the general hospital at Kingston, Georgia. A shell burst overhead, driving shrapnel into his right foot and shoulder. The hospital steward of his regiment, W. R. Grubb, threw him over a horse and led him to the rear. He was placed in an ambulance wagon and taken to the 1st Division Hospital of the 14th Corps, which was already full of wounded from the 23rd Corps. Tarbell's wounds were dressed by a doctor. On 30 May, he was placed in another ambulance wagon with others and started for Kingston. They slept on the road overnight. He arrived and was fed by another soldier, a Sergeant Kuenster of the 24th Illinois.

Three nurses helped him at Kingston, changing his dressing, but he saw no doctor.

Taylor, James E. "The Last Desperate Struggle: An Artist's Cedar Creek Battle Record." Edited by George Skoch. *Civil War Times Illustrated* 25 (December 1986): 32–39.

James Taylor was an artist working for *Frank Leslie's Illustrated Newspaper* during Sheridan's campaign in the Shenandoah Valley. He described and sketched the treatment of the wounded after the Battle of Cedar Creek. The churches in Middletown, Virginia were pressed into use as temporary hospitals. Operations took place in the church and the wounded then laid outside in the churchyard.

Taylor, Susie King. *Reminiscences of My Life in Camp with the 33rd United States Colored Troops, Late 1st S.C. Volunteers.* Boston: privately printed, 1902. Reprint. Louisville, KY: Lost Cause Press, 1958, 82 p.

The author was born a slave in Georgia in 1848. As a child in Savannah, she surreptitiously learned to read in a secret school run by a free black. In 1862, she escaped to St. Simon's Island, which, she noted, was full of blacks, but without many Yankees. She became a laundress, then a nurse, for the newly formed black regiment, the 1st South Carolina. The regiment made raids into Georgia, then invaded Jacksonville, Florida. The author was a nurse at the Jacksonville Hotel Hospital. She later visited the general hospital in Beaufort, South Carolina, and met Clara Barton. She does not give much detail of her nursing work, but her reminiscenes are full of interesting detail. Once the 1st South Carolina received mail that had been intended for the Confederate 1st South Carolina; it was sent to the Confederate regiment under flag of truce.

Taylor, William H. "Some Experiences of a Confederate Assistant Surgeon." In his *De Quibus: Discourses and Essays,* pp. 298–337. Richmond, VA: Bell Publishers, 1908.

Taylor describes his experiences as a regimental assistant surgeon many years later with humor. His relationship to his immediate superior, the regimental surgeon, is sarcastic. "All the surgeons I was acquainted with were social with their assistant surgeons. In quiet times they exhibited little pride of place, showing themselves patterns of equality and fraternity. But when a battle was imminent they were prone to become very lordly indeed, cavorting fussily around and ordering us assistant surgeons to move well up to the front, and giving us commands, which, if we had obeyed them to the letter, would have been the death of us; after which they retired, or to speak with accuracy, fled, to the shelter of their field hospitals." He also relates the famous story of the blue mass (mercury) in one pocket and in the other opium. If the soldier complained his bowels moved too freely, he got the opium, but if he was constipated, he got the mercury.

Tebault, Christopher H. "Hospitals of the Confederacy." *Southern Practitioner* 24 (1902): 499–509.

The author was a Confederate surgeon-in-charge of the general hospital in Griffin, Georgia. He states that every hospital bed was cleaned and dried in the sun every day. Patients were taken outside to sit in the shade during the cleaning. When a battle was expected, the medical director of the army (presumably the Army of Tennessee—Foard) notified the medical director of hospitals (Stout) to expect a deluge. Some general hospital doctors and male nurses would go to the battlefront in order to help evacuate the wounded. The author is writing in old age, and his memory betrays him. He must be incorrect when he says that "the general treatment of the Confederate Hospital Corps was aseptic, not antiseptic" and that it was more difficult to "sterilize" sponges than rags. His later practice presumably influenced his memory.

Thom, William Alexander. *"My Dear Brother": A Confederate Chronicle.* Edited by Catherine Thom Bartlett. Richmond, VA: Dietz Press, 1952, 224 p.

This book contains the letters of several people, two of whom were doctors. Although he had medical training, J. Pembroke Thom served in the Confederate States Army as a line officer, not as a surgeon. His brother, William Alexander Thom was a Confederate surgeon who, in two letters, tells the story of his 1864 trip from Richmond to Texas to inspect hospitals in the Trans-Mississippi Department. On the way back, he was captured and not released until after the end of the war.

Thompson, M. Jeff. *The Civil War Reminiscences of General M. Jeff Thompson.* Edited by Donal J. Stanton, G. F. Berquist, and P. C. Bowers, Dayton, OH: Morningside Press, 1988, 310 p.

The publication of this manuscript left by General Thompson shows the simplified way that guerrillas handled medical problems. The sick stayed home. Anyone wounded went home, sought help from friendly citizens, or was left behind for the Yankee surgeons to treat.

Thrall, Seneca B. "An Iowa Doctor in Blue: The Letters of Seneca B. Thrall, 1862–1864." Edited by Mildred Throne. *Iowa Journal of History* 58 (1960): 97–188.

Dr. Seneca B. Thrall, assistant surgeon of the 13th Iowa, wrote long letters home to his wife. Born in Ohio, he graduated from the medical faculty of the University of New York and moved to Ottumwa, Iowa, in 1856. He was with the 13th Iowa from late 1862 to early 1864; this regiment was part of the Iowa brigade, made up of 11th, 13th, 15th, and 16th Iowa. Thrall was present during the siege of Vicksburg. He has few medical comments except to note that his regiment was so healthy that the medical inspector thought that he was improperly filling out the medical reports.

Towle, Samuel K. "Notes of Practice in the U.S.A. General Hospital, Baton Rouge, La., during the Year 1863." *Boston Medical and Surgical Journal* 70 (1864): 49–60.

The author describes how he transformed the Louisiana Blind and Mute Asylum of Baton Rouge into the major general hospital for central Louisiana. His greatest problem was the removal of human waste from the hospital building.

Tripler, Charles S., and George C. Blackman. *Hand-book for the Military Surgeon.* Cincinnati: Robert Clarke and Co., 1861. Reprint. San Francisco: Norman Publishing, 1989, 121 p.

Tripler, a career army doctor, was Medical Director of the Army of the Potomac prior to his replacement by Letterman; Blackman was a colleague at the Medical College of Ohio in Cincinnati. This handbook was meant to instruct the military doctor in all the duties of his professional position. It included chapters on hygiene, dysentery, amputations, and wounds of the chest, abdomen, head, and arteries. The book went through several editions during the War; some editions add a 42-page appendix that reproduces official United States army medical forms.

Tripler, Eunice. *Eunice Tripler: Some Notes of Her Personal Recollections.* New York: Grafton Press, 1910, 184 p.

This book is by the widow of Charles S. Tripler, medical director of the Army of the Potomac, and later the United States Army representative to the American Medical Association. This is a very interesting and valuable work.

United States Navy Department, Bureau of Medicine and Surgery. *Instructions for the Government of the Medical Officers of the Navy of the United States.* Washington, DC: A. O. P. Nicholson, 1857, 43 p.

The introduction is by William Whelan, chief of the Bureau of Medicine and Surgery. The work contains numerous lists, such as the medical stores required on each ship and the names of all diseases (quite different from the Farr system). The diet list contains mainly staples that might be available on a long voyage; the only item containing much vitamin C is the potato. The examination for naval surgeons is given annually; it consists of a physical and a professional examination. All applicants for assistant surgeon must be between ages 21 and 25. All applicants for the position of surgeon must have served as an assistant surgeon for five years, with at least two years of sea duty.

United States Navy Department, Bureau of Medicine and Surgery. *Medical Essays: Compiled from Reports to the Bureau of Medicine and Surgery by Medical Officers of the U.S. Navy.* Washington, DC: Government Printing Office, 1872, 367 p.

The introduction to this work is by James C. Palmer. Ten reports include a very long work by Albert Leary Gihon entitled "Practical Suggestions in Naval Hygiene," two reports of yellow fever aboard naval vessels, and seven other short reports. None directly examine the medical problems of the recently concluded Civil War.

United States Navy Department, Naval War Records Office. *Official Records of the Union and Confederate Navies in the War of the Rebellion,* 30 vols. Washington, DC: Government Printing Office, 1894–1922.

A huge series of naval reports submitted during the War by both the Union and Confederate navies were compiled by two naval officers, Richard Rush and Robert H. Woods. This is the naval version of the much larger *Official Records of the Union and Confederate Armies* published by the Department of War. It includes some official reports from the Bureau of Medicine and Surgery. This series is often abbreviated in notes as *ORN,* for *Official Records, Naval.*

United States Sanitary Commission. *Hospital Transports: A Memoir of the Embarkation of the Sick and Wounded from the Penin-*

sula of Virginia in the Summer of 1862. Boston: Ticknor and Fields, 1863, 167.

This book is an important description of the Sanitary Commission steamers operating in support of the Army of the Potomac during the Peninsula campaign. The first section is a series of eyewitness reports by two Commission male officers and by two female nurses. The last section consists of the official correspondence of Frederick Law Olmsted.

United States Sanitary Commission. *The Sanitary Commission of the United States Army: A Succinct Narrative of its Works and Purposes.* New York: United States Sanitary Commission, 1864, 318 p.

An introduction on the origin of the United States Sanitary Commission emphasizes the role of Acting Surgeon General Robert C. Wood. The Commission organized soldier's homes, where the soldier could obtain food and rest; it maintained a hospital directory, so that civilians could find where their relatives are hospitalized; and it provided extra supplies to camp and to hospital. The book contains extracts from reports of inspectors that reveal immense detail. The inspection of 22 July 1863 revealed that Camp Letterman (amalgamated Union hospitals at Gettysburg) contained 13,050 wounded Union and 1,810 wounded Confederate soldiers, while Confederate physicians still maintained at Gettysburg 11 hospitals containing 5,452 wounded. This disjoined but important work contains all sorts of statistics: at the battle of Gettysburg, the Commission distributed $74,838.52 worth of goods, including 1,168 bottles of whiskey, 1,148 bottles of wine, 600 gallons of ale, 11,000 pounds of poultry and mutton, 12,500 pounds of milk, and 6,430 pounds of butter.

United States Surgeon General's Office. *Regulations for the Medical Department of the Army.* Washington, DC: A. O. P. Nicholson, Washington, 67 p. Revised edition. Washington, DC: Government Printing Office, 1861, 89 p. Reprint. Knoxville, TN: Bohemian Brigade Bookshop, 1989, 67 p.

This manual is a detailed statement of administrative duties of medical officers, including how to perform meterological observations. It includes blank forms. The edition of 1861 contains an introduction by Secretary of War Simon Cameron.

United States Surgeon General's Office. *Catalogue of the United States Army Medical Museum.* 3 vols. Washington, DC: Government Printing Office, 1866–67, 664 p., 136 p., 161 p. [Usually printed as 3 volumes in 2, but sometimes in 1.]

The catalog of the surgical section, prepared by A. A. Woodhull, contains many cases, surgical specimens, and woodcuts. "Private J. H.," Hospital Guards, Lovell General Hospital, Portsmouth Grove, Rhode Island, for example, while intoxicated, rushed at the sergeant of the guard and fell upon the point of the sergeant's sword; the specimen is the skull with broken sword point still within it. The second volume is the medical section, prepared by J. J. Woodward. "Private M.C.," 1st Michigan Cavalry, for example, suffered a pulmonary hemorrhage. While in Douglas Hospital, he lost over 60 pounds in two months and died on 27 August 1864; autopsy showed bright yellow tubercles throughout both lungs. The final volume is the catalog of the Microscopial Section, prepared by Edward Curtis.

United States Surgeon General's Office. *Photographs of Surgical Cases and Specimens Taken at the Army Medical Museum,* 7 vols. Washington, DC: Government Printing Office, 1866–72.

This work is an important series of photographs of wounded soldiers. Each picture is accompanied by a description of where and when the person was injured and a statement of his surgical therapy. The 181 photographs of the first four volumes are listed in the *Catalogue of the Army Medical Museum.* The seventh volume contains injuries from civilian life. George A. Otis was the compiler and William Bell the photographer.

United States Surgeon General's Office. *The Medical and Surgical History of the War of the Rebellion.* Washington, DC: Government Printing Office, 1875–85. Reprinted as *The Medical and Surgical History of the Civil War.* 12 vols. with 2 vol. index. Wilmington, NC: Broadfoot Publishing, 1990–92.

This huge series, begun by W. A. Hammond and carried to publication by J. K. Barnes, consisted of six huge books, divided into two volumes of three parts each.

Volume 1: Medical History, Part I, by J. J. Woodward consists of a summation of the medical returns for all major commands throughout the course of the War and the following year. Returns for black troops are separate. (726 pp.) This volume includes an appendix of excerpts from official reports by medical officers in the field. (369 pp.)

Volume 1: Medical History, Part II, by J. J. Woodward, concerns the great medical symptom of the war, diarrhea. Statistics from various commands and hospitals, including Confederate ones, are included. Fielding Garrison stated that this volume is the single most important historical work ever published on diarrhea and dysentery. (869 p.)

Volume 1: Medical History, Part III, by Charles Smart, is a collection of various subjects such as fevers, general hospitals, and disease among Confederates in Union prisons. (989 p.)

Volume 2: Surgical History, Part I, by George A. Otis, consists of a chronological list of military engagements with number of killed and wounded—as estimated by the Medical Bureau—followed by discussion of treatment of wounds of the head. (650 p.)

Volume 2: Surgical History, Part II, by George A. Otis, discusses wounds of the abdomen, pelvis, and arms. Many case reports are included. Surgeons performing operations are indexed. (1,024 p.)

Volume 2: Surgical History, Part III, by George A. Otis and D. L. Huntington discusses wounds of the legs, surgical complications such as secondary or late hemorrhage, anesthesia, official duties of ranking medical officers, and transportation of the sick and wounded. (986 p.)

Each part of the *Surgical Volume* has an index of operators and events but not of patients. The Broadfoot Publishing Company is reprinting this work with a complete index. This is the most important medical publication of the American Civil War.

United States War Department. *The War of the Rebellion: A Compilation of the Official Records of the Union and Confederate Armies,* 128 vols. Washington, DC: Government Printing Office, 1888.

This series of orders and reports, gathered under the direction of officers Robert N. Scott and Henry M. Lazelle, officially fills 128 volumes in four series. Many of these volumes consist of two or more parts, making a total of over 150 books each over 1,200 pages in length. The first series consists of contemporary communications relating to military campaigns. Many medical reports are included. General military reports contain many comments on the health of the troops. The fourth series contains many reports concerning the administration of the Medical Department of the Confederate States Army. This series is often abbreviated as *OR* in notes.

Upham, J. Baxter. "Hospital Notes and Memoranda." *Boston Medical and Surgical Journal* 68 (1863): 20–22.

The author reports he has become surgeon-in-charge of the United States Army hospital newly established at New Bern, North

Carolina. The hospital, named for Edward Stanley, Federal military governor of North Carolina, consists of several existing buildings in New Bern on the old Stanley Estate plus several newly built wooden pavilions. Upham states that each patient in the 520 beds will have "the quantum of air required by the Surgeon General in his circular of November 24th, 1862." The hospital was serviced by six doctors and two stewards, plus one nurse to every ten and one cook to every thirty patients. The nursing staff included Sisters of Mercy from the Convent of St. Catherine in New York.

Upham, J. Baxter. "Further Observations in Regard to the Cerebrospinal Affection Occurring in and around Newbern, N.C." *Boston Medical and Surgical Journal* 68 (1863): 311–17, 333–38.

Upham provides a very detailed description of the frightening epidemic that occurred among Union forces in New Bern, North Carolina. From the case descriptions of sudden onset, rapid progression, stiff neck, delirium, and in some cases petechial spots, it seems quite certain that this epidemic was meningococcal meningitis.

V

Vickery, Richard Swanton. "On the Duties of the Surgeon in Action." Edited by Albert Castel. *Civil War Times Illustrated* 17 (June 1978): 12–23.

Vickery was born in Ireland in 1831 and studied medicine in Dublin before coming to the United States in 1851. In 1860, he enrolled in the medical department of the University of Michigan. On 17 May 1861, he left medical school to become a private of the 2nd Michigan. He became assistant surgeon of the regiment on 8 August 1862 and participated in Second Manassas. He left the army in 1863 to return to medical school. His graduation thesis is herein published, slightly abridged. This essay gives an excellent survey of the Letterman system in action.

W

Wallace, William. "William Wallace's Civil War Letters." Edited by John O. Holzheuter. *Wisconsin Magazine of History* 57 (1973): 28–59 and 90–116.

William Wallace was born in 1830 in Ireland. He was a married farmer in Dodge County, Wisconsin, when he enlisted in the 3rd

Wisconsin. He was wounded at South Mountain in August of 1862 when a ball struck the little and ring fingers of his right hand (another ball went all the way through his hat). He was placed in a hospital in Christ Church, Alexandria, but had no care to his wound for some time. It healed with a ragged edge and the extraneous tissue was burned off with a caustic. He was helped by a visitor from the Wisconsin Aid Society. When the wounded from Antietam flooded the hospitals in the Washington area, he was sent to a convalescent camp. He was found to be suffering from rheumatic heart disease and received a medical discharge, dated 4 February 1863. But it is hard to keep an old war-horse in pasture. When his old regiment, the 3rd Wisconsin, was on leave in January 1864, his former colleagues convinced him to reenlist. He took part in the Georgia campaign, the taking of Atlanta, and the march to the sea. Despite the strain on his heart by this effort, he lived in Dodge County, Wisconsin, until his death in 1920 at age ninety.

Walton, Claiborne J. "One Continued Scene of Carnage: A Union Surgeon's View of War." *Civil War Times Illustrated* 15 (August 1976): 34–36.

Walton was surgeon of the 21st Kentucky (Union) and was an operating surgeon of his division after the Battle of Kennesaw Mountain. He estimated Union losses as 2,000, all occurring within a few minutes. The three operating tables of his division "were busy for several hours" after the battle. He was depressed when he wrote to his wife on 29 June 1864. "We have been on this campaign 56 days and it has been almost one continued scene of *carnage*," he wrote. "My hands are constantly steaped in blood. I have had them in blood and water so much that the nails are soft and tender. I have amputated limbs until it makes my heart ache to see a poor fellow coming in the ambulance to the hospital." He went on to conclude that "the horror of this war can never be half told."

Waring, Thomas Smith. "Confederate Surgeon: The Letters of Thomas Smith Waring, A South Carolina Planter-Physician at War." Edited by W. Curtis Worthington, Jr. *Journal of Confederate History* 2 (1989): 55–92.

Thomas Smith Waring was born in 1832 and graduated from the Medical College of South Carolina in 1853. Early in 1862, he became assistant surgeon of the 17th South Carolina. He was present at the Battle of Secessionville, near Charleston, on 18 June 1862. He received a scratch from shrapnel at the Battle of Second Manassas. His letters to his wife stop in 1863, but he survived the War and lived until 1901. These letters do not contain much material on his medical activities.

Warner, Adoniram J. "The Ordeal of Adoniram Judson Warner: His Minutes of South Mountain and Antietam." Edited by James B. Casey. *Civil War History* 28 (1982): 213–36.

An ordinary soldier gives his impressions of a complex operation performed two months after he was wounded at Antietam. The ball "was fast in the bone and took a great effort to get it out. The forceps the surgeon had were not strong enough. One pair broke and one bent in Dr. Brinton's hands and it became necessary to send to the Surgeon-General's office for a larger pair." The impressions of the surgeon for the same operation are given in the *Medical and Surgical History*, vol. 2, p. 329 (also p. 232). Warner survived and was later elected to the United States House of Representatives.

Warren, Edward. *An Epitome of Practical Surgery for Field and Hospital.* Richmond: West and Johnston, 1863. Reprint. San Francisco: Norman Publishing, 1989, 401 p.

Warren was a well-educated physician, a medical graduate of both the University of Virginia and of Jefferson Medical School. He obtained postgraduate experience under Jean-Martin Charcot in Paris. Though a native of North Carolina, he was on the faculty of the University of Maryland Medical School in 1861 and helped treat those injured in the riot associated with the passage of the 6th Massachusetts. He returned to his native state where he was made Surgeon General of state militia. He published this practical work, arranged according to illness or surgical procedure, in 1863. Although it bears a Richmond imprimature, it was published in Raleigh. The appendix presents surgical mortality in Richmond army hospitals during June and July of 1862.

Warren, Edward. *A Doctor's Experiences in Three Continents.* Baltimore: Cushings and Bailey, 1885, 613 p.

The author was on the faculty of the University of Maryland when the War began. He reports his shock when he saw the casualties brought to the university infirmary from the Baltimore riot at the passing of the 6th Massachusetts (Warren does not mention it, but William Hammond was in the infirmary at the same time). Warren was appointed surgeon-in-chief to the North Carolina Navy by the governor, but was at Charlottesville, Virginia, when the wounded from First Manassas poured into a system already full of soldiers sick with camp diseases such as measles. Warren gives an interesting description of his surgery on a soldier named Page. He was at New Bern, North Carolina, when it fell to Union forces. He has interesting observations of his next service: the examination of doctors to see if they had enough knowledge and skill to become or to remain Confederate army surgeons. He was with Lafayette Guild when the latter was made medical director of the Army of Northern Virginia. As the State Surgeon General of North Carolina in 1863, he supervised the vaccination of 70,000 people against the smallpox epidemic. He treated wounded Union and Confederate soldiers after the Battle of Bentonville in 1865. After the War, he practiced medicine in Egypt and in Paris.

Watkins, Sam R. *Co. Aytch, Maury Grays, First Tennessee Regiment; or, A Side Show of the Big Show.* Nashville, TN: Cumberland Presbyterian Publishing House, 1882, 223 p. Reprint. With an introduction by Bell Irwin Wiley. Jackson, TN: McCowat-Mercer Press, 1952, 231 p.

This is one of the best books written by a Confederate private. He only visited a hospital on one occasion—in Atlanta. "Great God! I get sick today," he wrote, "when I think of the agony, and suffering, and sickening stench and odor of dead and dying; of wounds and sloughing sores, caused by the deadly gangrene; of the groaning and wailing." At the rear of the building, he saw "a pile of arms and legs, rotting and decomposing; and, although I saw thousands of horrifying scenes during the war, yet today I have no recollection in my whole life, of ever seeing anything that I remember with more horror than that pile of legs and arms that had been cut off our soldiers." He saw a friend who had been shot during the attack of 22 July. He asked him if he were badly hurt and the wounded man, in reply, "pulled down the blanket, that was all. I get sick when I think of it. The lower part of his body was hanging to the upper part by a shred, and all of his entrails were lying on the cot with him, the bile and other excrements exuding from them, and they were full of maggots."

Watson, William. *Letters of a Civil War Surgeon.* Edited by Paul Fatout. West Lafayette, IN: Purdue University Studies, 1961, 110 p.

Watson was the surgeon of the 105th Pennsylvania, serving at Fredericksburg, Chancellorsville, and Gettysburg and during Grant's Virginia campaign. He was left behind with the wounded at the Battle of the Wilderness.

Webster, Warren. *An Address Delivered at the Inauguration of the*

Dale General Hospital, U.S.A., Worcester, Mass., February 22, 1865. Boston: Wright and Potter, 1865, 56 p.

The author was the surgeon-in-charge of DeCamp General Hospital, David's Island, New York Harbor. He presented the inaugural address at the general army hospital in Worcester, Massachusetts, named for William Johnson Dale, the surgeon general of the state militia of Massachusetts. The author reviewed the experiences of British and French forces during the Crimean War, attributing excessive deaths to medical disorganization. He contrasted the successful development of the Union Medical Bureau, especially its construction of general hospitals. At the beginning of the War, the United States Army had no general hospitals. At the time of this address, there were 195 with a bed capacity of 129,950.

Welch, Spencer Glasgow. *A Confederate Surgeon's Letters to His Wife*. New York: Neale Publishing Co., 1911. Reprint. Marietta, GA: Continental Book Company, 1954, 127 p.

Spencer Welch was the surgeon of the 13th South Carolina, McGowan's Brigade, Army of Northern Virginia. He sent his wife letters from Seven Days, Second Manassas, Antietam, Fredrickburg,, Chancellorsville, Gettysburg, the Wilderness, and Petersburg. He was a graduate of Jefferson Medical College, Philadelphia. Another surgeon who served with Welch was a son of former President Tyler; Welch criticized his gambling and drinking.

Wheelock, Julia Susan. *The Boys in White*. New York: Lange and Hillman, 1870, 268 p.

Julia Wheelock, later known as Mrs. Freeman, traveled from Ionia, Michigan, where she had been a school teacher, to Washington to care for her wounded brother, Orville Wheelock. Unfortunately he had died the day before her arrival. She determined to stay and work in the hospitals around Washington, treating other wounded soldiers as if they were her brother. She took a position with the Michigan Relief Association and disbursed food and clothing, to wounded from her home state initially, but later to the most needy. She kept a record of the hospital location of Michigan soldiers so that they could be found by relatives. At the beginning of the 1984 Virginia campaign, Miss Wheelock served at the field hospital of the 2nd Corps.

Wheelwright, Charles Henry. *Correspondence of Dr. Charles H. Wheelwright, Surgeon of the United States Navy*. Edited by Hildegarde B. Forbes. Boston: privately printed, 1958, 350 p.

Letters from the surgeon of the U.S.S. *San Jacinto* end in August 1862, when he died off Key West. [I was unable to read this work.]

Whetten, Harriet Douglas. "A Volunteer Nurse in the Civil War: The Letters and Diary of Harriet Douglas Whetten." Edited by Paul H. Hass. *Wisconsin Magazine of History* 48 (1965): 131–51 and 205–21.

Harriet Whetten of Staten Island, New York, became a volunteer nurse with the United States Sanitary Commission ships off the Virginia coast during the Peninsula Campaign. She was under the direct orders of Frederick Law Olmsted, but "reported" to Dorothea Dix at Yorktown. She met Miss Woolsey and the wife of Sanitary Commission treasurer George Templeton Strong. She was on the following ships at different times: *Knickerbocker, Wilson Small, Daniel Webster, Elm City,* and *Spaulding*. She also met Dr. John W. Draper, who was medical director on the St. Mark Floating Hospital. She gives detail of how many wounded were carried on each ship. Generally they were evacuated from bases such as West Point to Fort Monroe, or from Virginia to Washington, Philadelphia, or New York. Later in the War, Miss Whetten was in charge of nurses at Carter General Hospital in Washington. After the War, she became Mrs. Gamble of Intervale, New Hampshire.

Whitman, Walt. *The Wound Dresser*. New York: Small, Maynard, and Company, 1897, 200 p.

Whitman worked in Washington as a hospital volunteer, mainly in the Harewood Hospital, but also in the Armory Square Hospital. He brought the sick many small items to relieve their suffering; in one day, he brought different patients raspberry vinegar, a romance book, tobacco, and horehound candy. He was critical of the unfeeling medical care he observed. After less than a year's service as an unattached volunteer, he became depressed and left. He attributed his ill feeling to absorbing the hospital poison or "virus" given off by wounds (p. 196).

Whitman, Walt. *Walt Whitman and the Civil War*. Edited by Charles I. Glicksberg. Philadelphia: Unversity of Pennsylvania Press, 1933, 201 p.

This book contains all the material written by Whitman during the War including his diary for 1863 and his many letters to his mother. The editor has referenced every soldier to whom Whitman referred by name.

Wilkerson, Frank. "How Men Die in Battle." *Civil War Times Illustrated* 22 (April 1983): 16–19.

During the battles of the Wilderness and Spotsylvania in May of 1864, a Union army private made several observations about how men die after suffering a gunshot wound. Some are shot in the head and just keel over. He describes one who lived an hour after the head wound. "He did not speak. He simply lay on his back, and his broad chest rose and fell, slowly at first, and then faster and faster, and more and more feebly, until he was dead." One soldier struck in the head was knocked down, but then staggered to his feet; "with blood streaming from his head, he staggered aimlessly around in a circle, as sheep afflicted with grubs in the brain do." Confederate sharpshooters ended his misery.

When a soldier was struck in the body by a minie ball, he immediately tore off his clothing to examine the wound. Some would smile when they realized they were not badly wounded and might even get to go home. Others "would shrink back as from a blow and turn pale, as they realized the truth that they were mortally wounded." By 1864, soldiers could accurately judge a wound's prognosis. Wilkerson describes some soldiers with body wounds who knew they were bleeding internally; they gathered together and sat quietly. One told Wilkerson that he was smoking his last pipe of tobacco. Another tried to read a letter. The dying only called out to their mothers or described their homes when they became delirious. Wilkerson observed that, after death the face undergoes a series of changes of expression due to muscle contractions. "Sometimes the dead smile, again they stare with glassy eyes, and lolling tongues, and dreadfully distorted visages at you." One cannot tell from the facial expression whether the soldier died peacefully or in great terror.

Williams, Henry W. *A Practical Guide to the Study of Diseases of the Eye: Their Medical and Surgical Management.* Boston: Ticknor and Fields, 1862, 317 p.

Williams was born in Boston in 1821 and began the study of medicine at a relatively late age; he graduated from the medical department of Harvard University in 1849. He practiced ophthalmology in Boston for most of his life. A Civil War era physician wanting information about eye diseases would have referred to this work. In 1881, Williams wrote a much larger and more complete ophthalmology text, *The Diagnosis and Treatment of the Diseases of the Eye.*

Willson, George B. "Has the Brain Substance Any Sensibility?" *American Medical Times* 4 (1862): 204–5.

In the midst of war, scientific questions were examined. Willson, assistant surgeon of the 3rd Michigan, reported two cases—one with a skull injury from a saw accident and another from a gunshot wound—who flinched when he probed the brain substance. He therefore answers the title question affirmatively. [We now know that the brain only feels pain or touch when nerve endings are stimulated; there are no nerve endings in actual brain substance, but there are in the brain covering and in large blood vessels within the brain.] His military records in the National Archives spell Willson's name with one "l" and report that he resigned his commission on 15 June 1862.

Wilson, Legrand James. *The Confederate Soldier.* Fayetteville, AR: privately printed, 1902, 187 p. Reprint. Memphis, TN: Memphis State University Press, 1973, 213 p.

Wilson was born in 1836 and graduated from Jefferson Medical College in Philadelphia in 1859. In 1861, he became a line officer in the 1st Mississippi. He was apalled at the treatment given the many soldiers with measles; they were merely laid in a large tobacco barn, their fevers raged unchecked, and they often developed pneumonia. He urged the commanding officer to have them moved to individual homes where they could receive better nursing care from private families. He gradually shifted into the position of assistant surgeon, and, late in 1862, he passed the examination of the medical board and was appointed to the post of assistant surgeon of the 42nd Mississippi. The most interesting medical observations of this work are Wilson's activities at the Battle of Gettysburg. He was initially ordered to remain behind with the wounded but begged his way into a position supervising the terrible train of ambulance wagons carrying the wounded back into Virginia.

Wilson, Peter. "Peter Wilson in the Civil War." *Iowa Journal of History and Politics* 40 (1940): 153–203, 261–320, and 339–414.

Peter Wilson enlisted as a private in the 14th Iowa on 9 October 1861. He was captured in the Battle of Shiloh and released upon his oath that he would not serve in a military capacity until officially exchanged for a rebel in Yankee hands. Not knowing quite what to do with him, the Federal authorities made him a nurse, first in the regimental hospital of the 14th Iowa, then in the general hospital in Savannah, Tennessee, on the Tennessee River. There were about 2,000 patients in the hospital but about 1,500 could take care of themselves. Most were "worn out with diarrhea," but some were malingerers who "are playing off, as they call it, so as to shirk, and keep out of danger." Wilson was paid an additional $0.25 per day, bringing his pay to about $20 per month. He later became a ward master, supervising other male nurses. One of his duties involved digging graves.

Winchell, James. "Wounded and a Prisoner: A First-Person Account." *Civil War Times Illustrated* 4 (August 1965): 20–25.

The author, a private with Berdan's 1st United States Sharpshooters, received a splintering gunshot wound of the upper arm during the Battle of Gaines' Mill, 27 June 1862. About 500 wounded were left behind when the Union army retreated. The rebels treated him fairly well, but his arm became infested with maggots. He kept asking Union surgeons for help, but they replied that they would get to him "as soon as we get through with a few bad cases." His turn for amputation finally came but all the anesthetics had been used up. Winchell describes quite vividly the exact details of the amputation by Dr. Elisha M. White of the 20th Massachusetts.

The author was taken with the more seriously wounded Union soldiers to the Union prison hospital at Savage Station. He stayed there for about two weeks, eating terrible food and spitting drowned flies out of the water he drank. He was then taken by train to Richmond, across town by foot (until passersby saw his difficulty and arranged wagon transport), to another station, then by rail to Petersburg, where he was picked up by the Union steamer *Daniel Webster*. He was taken to Satterlee General Hospital in Philadelphia, where he thought that the medical students or, as he calls them, "the dude scholars," were eating the delicacies intended for the patients. It is interesting to compare the account of William Page, a Union physician at Savage Station.

Wittenmyer, Annie. *Under the Guns: A Woman's Reminiscences of the Civil War*. Boston: E. B. Stillings, 1895, 272 p.

Mrs. Wittenmyer helped care for the sick and wounded in the western theater. She was in Chattanooga during the Battle of Chickamauga and was present during the siege of Vicksburg. The book is a series of unconnected vignettes, not in chronological order.

Woodward, Joseph Janvier. *The Hospital Steward's Manual*. Philadelphia: J. B. Lippincott, 1862. Reprint. With an introduction by Ira M. Rutkow. San Francisco: Norman Publishing 1991, 324 p.

Assistant surgeon Woodward wrote this survey of a hospital steward's duties and submitted it to Surgeon General Hammond for his approval. Hammond appointed a board, consisting of Surgeons Joseph K. Barnes and Joseph R. Smith, who concluded that the work was "written in strict accordance with the regulations of the army and the customs of the service." Hammond, therefore, made this an offical military medical manual. The book spells out the status of all hospital personnel. The hospital steward is a noncommissioned officer at the same rank as an ordnance sergeant; in 1861 received $22 per month, raised the next year to $30. He wore an enlisted man's uniform with crimson trim, a red sash, and a chevron on each arm marked by a yellow caduceus. Enlisted men could be detailed as hospital attendants, designated as cooks or nurses. They received, in addition to their regular pay, an extra $0.25 per day. Civilians could be hired as similar attendants and were paid $20.50 per month. Female nurses received $0.40 per day plus rations and room. "Women wishing employment as nurses must apply to Miss Dix or to her authorized agents," but nuns were excepted. Laundresses, usually the wives of soldiers, were paid $6 per month plus rations. The manual is full of rules of hospital life, such as: latrines "should never be dug in the neighborhood of wells" (p. 111).

Woodward, Joseph Janvier. *Outline of the Chief Camp Diseases of the United States Armies as Observed during the Present War.* Philadelphia: J. B. Lippincott, 1863. Reprint. With an introduction by Saul Jarcho. New York: Hafner, 1964. Reprint. San Francisco: Norman Publishing, 1991, 364 p.

Woodward served with the Surgeon General's Office. In this book, he writes about camp fevers and includes statistics from the first year of the War. He concluded that measles could occur only once in each individual and was best treated conservatively. In this work, Woodward introduced the term "typho-malarial fever" for a person with a prolonged, intermittent fever who developed pneumonia.

Woodward, Joseph Janvier. *Report on Epidemic Cholera in the Army of the United States During the Year 1866.* Washington, DC: GPO, 1867, 65 p.

Woodward constructed this report for Surgeon General Barnes, who issued it as Circular Number 5 of 4 May 1867. He traced the cholera epidemic as it traveled through army posts in the last half of 1866. Interesting statistics are given for white troops in thirty-one posts in the United States and Nicaragua and for colored troops in twelve locations, all in the southern United States. These garrisons averaged 12,789 soldiers during the last half of 1866. Of these, 2,708 developed cholera and 1,207 died. Therefore, these posts lost about 10 percent of their complement due to cholera.

Woodward does not observe that the military mortality would have been frightful if this epidemic had struck one year earlier.

Woolsey, Jane S. *Hospital Days*. New York: Van Nostrand, 1870, 182 p.

This book covers the author's services as a nurse and matron with the Fairfax Seminary Hospital, Alexandria, Virginia, under the direction of Dr. David P. Smith. Her sister, Georgeanna, was with her for a period, but, during the 1864 Virginia campaign, she served with the hospital support system of the Army of the Potomac. The author describes the difficulties of receiving large numbers of sick and wounded; one of the largest influxes of sick occurred after the great victory march in Washington in May of 1865.

Wormeley, Katherine Prescott. *The Cruel Side of War with the Army of the Potomac*. Boston: Ticknor, 1889, 207 p.

The author was appointed by the Sanitary Commission to accompany ships hired to transport the sick and wounded during the Peninsula campaign. She made several trips from New York City or Newport, Rhode Island, to and from White House, Harrison's Landing, or Fortress Monroe. She generally made herself useful, performing such tasks as writing letters for soldiers, from both North and South, who were too weak to write for themselves. She describes the inspection visit of Henry J. Bigelow just prior to the appointment of Hammond as surgeon general. Her views of typhoid fever are interesting: "You are not to be alarmed by the word, typhoid, which I foresee will occur on every page of my letters, nearly all our sick cases being that or running into that," she reassured her family. "The idea of infection is simply absurd. The ventilation of these ships is excellent; besides, people employed in such a variety of work and in high health and spirits are not liable to infection."

Worsham, John H. *One of Jackson's Foot Cavalry*. New York: Neale Publishing Company, 1912, 353 p.

This detailed history of one company, Company F of the 21st Virginia, gives many interesting medical details. Three privates were physicians, and they all became medical officers, transferring to other regiments. The company suffered twenty-six combat deaths and twenty-four soldiers captured. During the course of the War, nine soldiers were discharged because of wounds (of a total of twenty-seven wounded), and thirteen were discharged from the army because of chronic illness (chronic rheumatism, chronic diarrhea, chronic typhoid, coronary artery disease, edema of the legs, epilepsy, and idiocy). Three soldiers died of disease. Six members of the company were reassigned as hospital stewards and three received special duty for medical reasons (one as guard and two as clerks). Seven soldiers remained on the rolls of F Company, but were in Richmond general hospitals for many months.

Wyeth, John A. *With Sabre and Scalpel.* New York: Harper, 1914, 535 p.

Wyeth was an enlisted soldier in the Confederate States Army. He was with Morgan in Kentucky and was present at the Battle of Chickamauga. After the War he attended medical school in New York. This work contains virtually nothing on Confederate medicine.

Y

Yarrow, Henry Crecy. "Personal Recollections of Some Old Medical Officers." *Military Surgeon* 60 (1927): 73–76, 171–75, 449–55, 588–93.

The author offers interesting personal evaluations of some medical officers of the regular army, including George Otis, John Randolph, Joseph Janvier Woodward, and John Shaw Billings. William A. Hammond inspected the author's hospital at Broad and Cherry Streets, Philadelphia: "a more arrogant or pompous individual had never visited the hospital." The author states that "during the time that he was Surgeon General those who knew him rarely found him anything but captious, irritable and pompous." Yarrow relates a story about Horace Raquet Wirtz, the Medical Director of Union forces in the Department of the South on Hilton Head Island, South Carolina. Asked if he remembered that his female hospital matron had been killed, swept overboard from a ship, he replied seriously: "I expect to burn in hell for that."

SECONDARY SOURCES

A

Abolins, Andrea. "Oh, Dem Bones, Dem Dry Bones." *Civil War Times Illustrated* 30 (September 1991): 41.

Several small fragments of hair and bone from President Lincoln's head wound were placed in the Army Medical Museum in 1865. The name of the Museum has changed to the National Museum of Health and Medicine, but Lincoln's specimens are still there. Dr. Darwin Prockop has proposed to analyze a small portion of this tissue by modern DNA techniques to determine if Lincoln suffered from the unusual disorder known as Marfan's syndrome. Despite its puerile title, this brief article is interesting and accurate. Museum officials worried that revelations about Lincoln's health might contradict the slain president's posthumous right to privacy. A special committee on ethics has approved the study, now under way. The author of this article does not reveal her opinion about Lincoln and Marfan. This reviewer does not have the expertise to judge the value of the proposed DNA analysis, but confidently predicts that Lincoln did not have Marfan's syndrome.

Ackerknecht, Erwin H. *Malaria in the Upper Mississippi Valley, 1760–1900*. Baltimore: Johns Hopkins Press, 1945, 142 p.

Malaria was common in the upper Mississippi region, from Illinois to Minnesota and Iowa, during the period of initial settlement. The author hypothesizes that the early settlers produced changes in natural water drainage, the stagnant water increased the mosquito population, and the greater number of mosquitos spread the malarial parasite. As the area became more settled, this process was reversed and malaria disappeared as a public health problem. The decline in the incidence of malaria was not due to increased use of quinine.

Ackerknecht, Erwin H. "Anticontagionism between 1821 and 1867." *Bulletin of the History of Medicine* 22 (1948): 562–93.

The idea that a disease could spread directly from one person to another by a mysterious process called contagion was accepted by the Hebrew writers of the Old Testament and the quarantines of the fifteenth century were based upon it. But, by the early nineteenth century, according to Ackerknecht, the opposing doctrine of anti-contagionism became popular throughout Europe. Epidemics in Europe and among European armies throughout the world throughout the nineteenth century revived the ideas of contagion and set the stage for the discoveries of bacteriology. The experiences and writings of American doctors from the Civil War period are not mentioned.

Adams, George W. "Confederate Medicine." *Journal of Southern History* 6 (1940): 151–66.

The article begins with the assertion that "the Civil War was fought in the very last years of the medical middle ages" and ends with a statement that much loss of life among Confederate forces could have been saved by proper application of existing medical knowledge. "The medical theory and medical practice of the time were both faulty," Adams concludes, "but they were both good enough to have saved perhaps half the lives lost had the fates been kinder." He points to decreased resistance to disease because of exposure (too few blankets) and because of poor diet. The Confederates failed to emphasize the truism that "personal and camp cleanliness are high among the military virtues." Adams does not examine the hypothesis that if these lives had been saved or if the Confederate armies had been healthier, the War might have taken a different course.

Adams, George W. *Doctors in Blue: The Medical History of the Union Army in the Civil War.* New York: Henry Schuman, 1952. Reprint. Dayton, OH: Morningside Press, 1985, 253 p.

The standard classic on medical care in the Union army has chapters on hospitals, nurses, ambulances, and diseases.

Adams, George W. "Caring for the Men." In *The Image of War, 1861–1865,* edited by William C. Davis. vol. 4, pp. 231–74. Garden City, NY: Doubleday, 1983.

A brief description of medical care, North and South, accompanies a magnificent set of photographs. The images vary from distant views of hospitals to a grimy mass of discarded human legs.

Allen, Phyllis. "Etiological Theory in America prior to the Civil

War." *Journal of the History of Medicine and Allied Sciences* 2 (1947): 489–520.

The importation of the French method of postmortem examination in the 1820s led to increased skill in clinical diagnosis, particularly a differentiation of the many different disorders subsumed under the heading of fever. A renewed interest in etiology followed with special attention to how disease could spread from one person to another.

Allen, Sue. "Dr. Requa's Gun: Odd Looking, Fast Shooting, Obsolete." *Civil War Times Illustrated* 27 (February 1989): 28–33.

Dr. Josephus Requa was a dentist in Rochester, New York. He helped to develop a multibarrel weapon, a forerunner of the machine gun. It was used by Federal forces at the sieges of Port Hudson and Fort Wagner with some good effect.

Anderson, Donald Lee, and Godfrey T. Anderson. "Nostalgia and Malingering in the Military during the Civil War." *Perspectives in Biology and Medicine* 28 (1984): 156–66.

This article evaluates two unrelated diagnoses or conditions, nostalgia (excessive homesickness) and malingering, mainly from the Union viewpoint.

Anderson, Ella. "Crazy Bet Van Lew was General Grant's Eyes and Ears in Richmond." *America's Civil War* 4 (July 1991): 8.

This article briefly surveys the wartime career of Elizabeth L. Van Lew, a citizen of Richmond who remained loyal to the Union. While the substance of the report concerns her activities as a spy, she visited wounded Union officers in Libby prison and persuaded the Confederate doctors to transfer them to Confederate hospitals.

Andrews, Matthew Page. *The Women of the South in War Times.* Baltimore: Norman Remington Co., 1920, 466 p.

This book contains brief descriptions of several leading Southern women, including Sally Tompkins and several nurses. Mrs. Ella K. Newsome (referred to by the name of her second, postwar husband, Trader) is called the "Florence Nightingale of the South." The book includes the diary of Judith Brockenbrough McGuire, wife of John P. McGuire, principal of the Episcopal High School near Alexandria, Virginia. Her diary, running from 4 May 1861 to 4 May 1865, contains some nursing observations from Lynchburg and Richmond.

Ashburn, Percy M. *A History of the Medical Department of the U.S. Army.* Boston: Houghton Mifflin, 1929, 448 p.

This general history by an army medical officer contains a large section on the Civil War.

Austerman, Wayne. "Maynard: A Carbine Made in Massachusetts, the Favorite of Southern Soldiers." *Civil War Times Illustrated* 25 (April 1986): 42.

Dr. Edward Maynard was trained as a physician and practiced dental surgery. He had attended West Point and became interested in firearm technology. He used his expertise with dental tools to develop a rifle named after him.

Austin, Anne L. *The Woolsey Sisters of New York: A Family's Involvement in the Civil War and a New Profession, 1860–1900.* Philadelphia: American Philosophical Society, 1917, 189 p.

This excellent book discusses the lives of the seven daughters of Charles William and Jane Eliza Newton Woolsey. George Anna Muirson Woolsey, known as Georgeanna or Georgy, and Eliza Newton Woolsey served as nurses at hospitals in the Washington area and on transports in the James river during the Peninsula campaign. Georgy and her mother helped at Camp Letterman after the Battle of Gettysburg. Two other sisters were pioneers in the education of female nurses in New York in the 1870s.

B

Baird, Nancy Disher. "The Yellow Fever Plot." *Civil War Times Illustrated* 13 (November 1974): 16–23.

Yellow fever broke out in Bermuda in April of 1864. A Confederate physician, Luke Pryor Blackburn of Kentucky, was sent to the island, a center for blockade running, and helped treat yellow fever patients. After the War, Blackburn was accused of taking clothing and bedding from yellow fever patients and smuggling this material into several Northern cities. It was charged that the doctor intended to distribute the clothing in order to spread yellow fever to the unsuspecting populace, producing a horrible epidemic that would paralyze the Northern war effort. A hearing was held in Canada, where the plot supposedly originated, and some witnesses testified; no full trial with cross-examination ever occurred. After the War, Dr. Blackburn returned to the practice of medicine and eventually became governor of Kentucky. The author comes to no definite conclusion about his guilt; the evidence is circumstantial but suggestive. Today, we know that the virus of yellow fever is carried from one victim to another only by mosquitoes and that this plot, which involved clothing stored for prolonged periods, could not have succeeded. Baird concludes that even if Southern agents had produced an epidemic in Northern cities, "it is doubtful that even yellow fever could have weakened the Union sufficiently to alter the outcome" of the War.

Baird, Nancy Disher. *David Wendell Yandell: Physician of Old Louisville*. Lexington: University Press of Kentucky, 1978, 116 p.

This biography of Yandell includes one chapter on his four years with the Confederate Army.

Baird, Nancy Disher. "There Is No Sunday in the Army: Civil War Letters of Lunsford P. Yandell, 1861–62." *Filson Club Historical Quarterly* 53 (1979): 317–27.

Lunsford P. Yandell, Jr. (1837–84) was a brother of David Wendell Yandell (1826–98). He graduated from the Louisville Medical Institute, founded by his father, in 1857 and two years later moved to Memphis, where he was on the faculty of the Memphis Medical College. He served as assistant surgeon with the 4th Tennessee. He observed that "disease in camp is different from disease in town. I have heretofore been almost an anti-calomel doctor, but the cases which we have to deal with here demand the use of mercurials." His unit was stationed along the Mississippi, where they frequently came under fire from Yankee gunboats. On 7 November 1861, Yandell and the 4th Tennessee crossed the Mississippi to help defend Belmont, Missouri. He treated many wounded, both Confederate and Federal. He accompanied the Federal wounded under flag of truce when they were taken to General Grant at Cairo, Illinois. Later in the War, he was medical inspector for General Hardee.

Baker, Nina Brown. *Cyclone in Calico: The Story of Mary Ann Bickerdyke*. Boston: Little, Brown, 1952, 278 p.

This work is the standard biography of Mother Bickerdyke from Galesburg, Illinois, who acted as a Union nurse. She was at Corinth during the battle of 3 October, 1862 and was present at the siege of Vicksburg and during the Atlanta Campaign. The biographer says she was "a thorn in the side" of the doctor in charge of the Memphis hospitals, Dr. B. J. D. Irwin. When she thought a hospital too dirty, she undertook a nonstop cleaning operation that she called a "cyclone clean-up," hence the nickname she earned during the War, "the cyclone in calico."

Barton, George. *Angels of the Battlefield: A History of the Labors of the Catholic Sisterhoods in the Late Civil War.* Philadelphia: Catholic Art Publishing Co., 1897, 302 p.

Prior to the War, four different orders had nursing experience. They were the Sisters of Charity, the Sisters of Mercy, the Sisters of St. Joseph, and the Sisters of the Holy Cross. The Sisters of Charity had three groups: the Sisters of Charity of Nazareth, Kentucky, the Cornette Sisters of Emmitsburg, Maryland (noted for their white caps), and the Mother Seton Sisters (noted for their black caps). This work, based mainly upon personal interviews, made difficult by "the genuine humility so characteristic of the Sisters," devotes several chapters to each of these orders. Service for both sides in the War is covered, but the emphasis is upon nursing for the North.

After the Battle of Shiloh, Dr. Blackmun and three Sisters from Cincinnati went to the battle site and served aboard hospital ships in the Tennessee River. Sister Anthony helped Dr. Blackmum perform surgery. Walter F. Atlee, a leading Philadelphia physician had interviews with Hammond and Stanton in order to obtain permission to use Sisters as nursing personnel at the huge Satterlee Hospital of West Philadelphia. On 9 June 1862, the hospital was opened with sixty Sisters of Charity. The chief nurse, Sister Mary Gonzaga, made rounds late at night, silently moving from bed to bed. The Sisters of Mercy ran the nursing services on the hospital ship, *Empress,* and were also at the Stanton Hospital in Washington. The Sisters of Charity from Emmitsburg, accompanied by Father Burlando, traveled to the Peninsula to nurse the wounded and sick at the base hospital at the White House. Sister M. Collette O'Connor was chief nurse at the Douglas Hospital in Washington; she died there of typhoid fever on 16 July 1864.

Many Sisters provided nursing after the Battle of Gettysburg. Several Sisters of Charity, again accompanied by Father Burlando, set up in the Methodist church in the town. This led to a humorous exchange, when a soldier issuing supplies at the supply wagon asked a Sister if she were from the Catholic church; she replied: "No, I am from the Methodist Church." The major point of the book concerns how the courageous War service of Catholic Sisters accelerated their acceptance as valuable members of society.

Bassham, Ben. "Through a Mist of Powder and Excitement: A Southern Artist at Shiloh." *Tennessee Historical Quarterly* 47 (1988): 131–41.

Conrad Wise Chapman became famous after the War for his paintings of wartime scenes, especially scenes of Charleston harbor. This article concerns his early Confederate service as a private with the 3rd Kentucky, part of the Orphan Brigade. Of major medical interest is the wound he received at Shiloh, where he was struck by a spent ball that penetrated his forehead and went halfway around his head under his scalp. He bled profusely at first until his wound was dressed by the regimental surgeon. He had to walk most of the way to Corinth. He was evacuated to the Overton Hospital in Memphis by train, but experienced a derailment. He later returned to his unit, stationed in Memphis, but he became ill "from the city's contaminated water."

Baxley, Haughton. "Surgeons of the Confederacy: Edward Warren of North Carolina." *Confederate Veteran* 34 (1926): 172–73.

Dr. Warren was at the Charlottesville Hospital; he was briefly medical inspector of the Army of Northern Virginia. After the War he served in the medical department of the Egyptian Army. Later he obtained license to practice medicine in Paris and died in that city.

Bayne-Jones, Stanhope. *The Evolution of Preventive Medicine in the United States Army, 1607–1939.* Washington, DC: Government Printing Office, 1968, 255 p.

This book includes a useful summary of preventive medicine in the Union army and praises Hammond. The author was the grandson of Joseph Jones, but Confederate medical activities are not mentioned.

Beshoar, Barron B. *Hippocrates in a Red Vest: The Biography of a Frontier Doctor.* Palo Alto, CA: American West Publishing Co., 1973, 352 p.

Michael Beshoar, grandfather of the author, was from Pennsylvania and of German background. After graduation in medicine from the University of Michigan, he set up practice in a small town in northeastern Arkansas. When the War broke out, he, like his friends and neighbors, joined the Confederate army. He was surgeon of the 7th Arkansas and operated extensively after the Battle of Shiloh. Captured with Jeff Thompson in Arkansas, he eventually took the oath of allegiance and was released so that he could set up a private practice in Ironton, Missouri. He later joined the Union army as an acting assistant surgeon, serving first in St. Louis and then at Fort Kearny on the frontier. The fort was garrisoned by the 3rd United States Volunteers, made up of Confederate prisoners who joined the Union army on condition that they would serve against Indians but never against Confederates. They were called "galvanized Yankees." Most of this very interesting book concerns Beshoar's life on the frontier after the War.

Black, Robert C., III. *The Railroads of the Confederacy.* Chapel Hill: University of North Carolina Press, 1952, 360 p.

This is the definitive work on the Confederate railroad network. There were difficulties from the beginning because the rails were of different gauge, requiring passengers and goods to be transferred from one rail system to another. The major problem, however, was the lack of facilities and expertise to build and repair rails, engines, and cars. As the War progressed, wear and tear—even more than enemy action—produced a chronic deterioration of the Confederate rail network. The author does not specifically mention medical problems, but the information in this work illuminates the medical transportation difficulties that produced much suffering for the sick and wounded.

Blaisdell, F. William. "Medical Advances during the Civil War." *Archives of Surgery* 123 (1988): 1045–50.

The medical and surgical accomplishments of the Civil War era have been relatively unappreciated because of comparison to modern standards. These accomplishments are listed: (1) The publication of the *Medical and Surgical History of the War of the Rebellion,* "the first major academic accomplishment of U.S. medicine"; (2) the development of a system for handling mass casualties that set the pattern for World War I; (3) the pavilion style of hospital construction, copied by civilian hospitals for seventy-five years; (4) surgeons learned the importance of early operation after major trauma; (5) physicians learned that hygiene and sanitation prevented many diseases; (6) the introduction of female nurses on a large scale; (7) the military standards of army physicians became national medical standards; and (8) the United States Sanitary Commission set the pattern for the development of the American Red Cross.

Blanton, Wyndham B. *Medicine in Virginia in the Nineteenth Century.* Richmond: Garrett and Massie, 1933, 449 p.

This classic work devotes a long section to the Civil War. It contains a list of Virginia physicians who served the Confederate States Army or Navy.

Blaser, Martin J., Joy G. Wells, Roger A. Feldman, Robert A. Pollard, and James R. Allen. "Campylobacter Enteritis in the United States." *Annals of Internal Medicine* 98 (1983): 360–65.

This modern study of diarrhea evaluated patients admitted to the hospital because of this symptom. Most had no cause for the diarrhea determined, but many had a positive stool culture for bacteria. The most common bacterial causes were Campylobacter, followed by Salmonella and Shigella. In southern states, Shigella was more common than either of the other two organisms. Patients with Campylobacter diarrhea were more likely to complain of tenesmus [during the Civil War, soldiers with diarrhea and tenesmus received the diagnosis of dysentery]. Bacterial diarrhea was often associated with fever. One can assume that these same organisms caused diarrhea during the Civil War.

Blochman, Lawrence G. *Doctor Squibb: Life and Times of a Rugged Idealist.* New York: Simon and Schuster, 1958, 371 p.

The Civil War transformed Squibb's drug operation from a personal chemist shop to a huge industry.

Blustein, Bonnie Ellen. "To Increase the Efficiency of the Medical Department." *Civil War History* 33 (1987): 22–41.

The War modernized medicine by increasing the authority of a medical elite over medical practice, by requiring the administration of a standardized test to all physicians, and by demonstrating the value of medical science. The author concludes that "the Civil War experience was critically important in setting not only the pace but the pattern of civilian medical science and practice in the last third of the century."

Bollet, Alfred Jay. "To Care for Him That Has Borne the Battle: A Medical History of the Civil War." *Medical Times* 117 (April 1989): 121–26; (May 1989): 101–8; (October 1989): 74–80.

The author, a specialist in internal medicine, provides an overview of the medical problems of the War. He is especially strong in teasing modern diseases from the various obscure diagnoses of the nineteenth century. This essay may contain the best analysis of the enteric diseases, diarrhea and dysentery.

Bollet, Alfred Jay. "Scurvy, Sprue, and Starvation: Major Nutritional Deficiency Syndromes During the Civil War." *Medical Times* 117 (November 1989): 69–74; 118 (June 1990): 39–44.

The only nutritional disease recognized by doctors during the War was scurvy. The scorbutic tendency (subclinical scurvy) produced lassitude and depression in large numbers of soldiers; it may have been a major factor in Union failure during the campaign on the Peninsula in 1862. Other nutritional syndromes that may have occurred are night blindness due to vitamin A deficiency and the sprue syndrome due to folate deficiency.

Boritt, Gabor S., and Adam Boritt. "Lincoln and the Marfan Syndrome: The Medical Diagnosis of a Historical Figure." *Civil War History* 29 (1983): 212–19.

This article combines the medical and historical talents of two brothers. Adam Boritt is a pathologist; he examines the pros and cons of the diagnosis of Marfan's syndrome and concludes that Lincoln did not suffer from that disorder. Gabor Boritt is a historian; he examines the subsconscious motivations of people making the diagnosis of Marfan's syndrome and concludes that this diagnosis is an aspect of Lincoln mythology. "Lincoln the Marfan" is a version of the old idea of "Lincoln the Illegitimate."

Boyd, Mark F. "An Historical Sketch of the Prevalence of Malaria in North America. *American Journal of Tropical Medicine* 21 (1941): 223–44.

Malaria was probably not present in the New World prior to the arrival of Europeans. In the United States, malaria tended to follow the frontier. Boyd hypothesizes that increased human habitation changed drainage patterns, leading to a marked increase in the number of mosquitoes. This was especially true during the digging of the Erie Canal. With the regularization of drainage patterns, malaria decreased in the North, but it remained a problem in the "more primitive" South. Boyd has a short section on malaria during the Civil War, largely taken from the *Medical and Surgical History*. Malaria became a greater problem during and following the War in the South because of many new people with no immunity to the disorder and because the mosquito population increased following the general disorganization of farming patterns.

Boyden, Anna L. *Echoes from Hospital: A Record of Mrs. Rebecca R. Pomroy's Experience in War-Times*. Boston: D. Lothrop, 1884, 250 p.

Pomroy was selected as a nurse for Georgetown Hospital by Dorothea Dix early in the War. She argued with the Catholic fathers about theology. She visited Lincoln at the White House.

Breeden, James O. "Andersonville: A Southern Surgeon's Story." *Bulletin of the History of Medicine* 47 (1973): 317–43.

Joseph Jones wrote a "full and frank" report of medical conditions at Andersonville Prison to the Confederate surgeon general. Accompanied by his secretary, Louis Manigault, Jones arrived at the prison in September 1864. He surveyed the hospital and dead house (morgue), but had to get special permission from General Winder in order to enter the prison grounds. He estimated 5,000 seriously ill with 90 to 130 deaths per day. He noted the horrible stench of human feces from the stockade. The report gives hospital statistics, including the number of prisoners "returned to duty" (i.e., returned to the stockade). The illness rate among the guards was quite high. The worst diseases: diarrhea/dysentery and scurvy. Portions of the report were used in the trial of the prison commander, Heinrich Wirz.

Breeden, James O. *Joseph Jones, M.D.: Scientist of the Old South.* Lexington: University Press of Kentucky, 1975, 293 p.

This is an excellent biography of Joseph Jones with a large section on his Civil War experiences. Late in the War, he was sent by the surgeon general to survey the medical situation in Georgia, Alabama, and Mississippi.

Breeden, James O. "A Medical History of the Later Stages of the Atlanta Campaign." *Journal of Southern History* 35 (1969): 31–59.

This article evaluates medical statistics for July and August of 1864. The Confederate information is taken from the Jones papers at Tulane and the Union from the *Medical and Surgical History.* More malaria occurred in Union forces, but fewer deaths from malaria. Diarrhea/dysentery was also more common among the Union soldiers. Measles caused 1,400 hospitalizations among Confederates, but only 14 in the Union army. The Confederacy experienced a greater number of gunshot wounds, but a lower mortality from this source. Of the 80,000 Confederates hospitalized during these two months, only 2 percent died; however, only 20 percent returned to duty (the others being discharged, furloughed, or evacuated).

Breeden, James O. "States-Rights Medicine in the Old South." *New York Academy of Medicine Bulletin* 52 (1976): 348–72.

As part of the growing feeling of nationalism in the South in the 1850s, Southern physicians developed a series of ideas concerning local medical care and problems. In the first place, blacks experienced diseases differently than whites. In the second place, Southern diseases were different than Northern ones. Therefore, many

Southern physicians thought that the South should develop its own medical schools and its own medical science and attempt to dissociate itself from Northern medicine. Even an economic factor was present in this doctrine of "states-rights medicine." Each year, one-half of the 2,500 Southern youth studying medicine went to Northern cities, particularly Philadelphia, to study. They spent upwards of one-half million Southern dollars in the North. Breeden gives statistics showing markedly increased enrollments in Southern medical schools in the late 1850s.

Breeden, James O. "Oscar Lieber: Southern Scientist, Southern Patriot." *Civil War History* 36 (1990): 226–49.

Oscar Lieber was a geologist who went with the Confederacy while his father, Francis Lieber, remained loyal to the Union. He was wounded in the battles around Richmond in 1862 and died in a Richmond hospital.

Bres, P. L. J. "A Century of Progress Combatting Yellow Fever." *Bulletin of the World Health Organization* 64 (1986): 775–86.

Yellow fever could strike terror into coastal populations of the Americas throughout the eighteenth and nineteenth centuries. The last major American epidemic was in the Mississippi valley in 1878, producing 13,000 cases and 5,000 deaths. The article emphasizes how the yellow fever virus and its transmission by mosquito were discovered early in the twentieth century.

Brewer, James H. *The Confederate Negro: Virginia's Craftsmen and Military Laborers, 1861–1865*. Durham, NC: Duke University Press, 1969, 212 p.

From detailed study of hospital records, the author has culled out the activities of black workers at many Confederate military hospitals in Virginia. Chimborazo Hospital, Richmond, for example, at the beginning of 1863 employed 166 detailed white soldiers, 25 white woman matrons, 264 male black nurses, 54 black cooks, and 123 female black laundry workers.

Brieger, Gert H. "Therapeutic Conflicts and the American Medical Profession in the 1860s." *Bulletin of the History of Medicine* 41 (1967): 215–22.

This article reviews the order of Surgeon General Hammond that removed calomel from the list of army medicines. The maelstorm that followed is seen as a clash between two medical philsophies: Nature (self-limited disease, therapeutic scepticism) and Art (intervention). Hammond, Oliver Wendell Holmes, Austin Flint, Stephen Smith, and Jacob Bigelow represented the former school.

Briggs, Walter DeBlois. *Charles Edward Briggs: Civil War Surgeon in a Colored Regiment.* Berkeley: University of California, 1960, 166 p.

Charles Edward Briggs (1833–94) graduated from Harvard Medical School in 1856. After two years as assistant surgeon with the 24th Massachusetts, he was promoted to surgeon with the 54th Massachusetts, a regiment of black troops. This regiment served on the Carolina coast. This brief work by the doctor's grandson contains a few medical observations.

Brings, Hans A. "Navy Medicine Comes Ashore: Establishing the First Permanent U.S. Navy Hospital." *Journal of the History of Medicine and Allied Sciences* 41 (1986): 257–92.

This article emphasizes naval medicine in the early years of the Republic. Before 1828, a surgeon went off-pay when his ship was decommissioned. The Navy Department established a Bureau of Medicine and Surgery only in 1842.

Brockett, Linus Pierpont. *The Camp, the Battlefield and the Hospital; or, Lights and Shadows of the Great Rebellion.* Philadelphia: National Publishing Co., 1866. Reprint. *Battlefield and Hospital; or, Lights and Shadows of the Great Rebellion.* Philadelphia: Hubbard Brothers, 1888, 512 p.

Many brief stories about spies, rescues, and "daring enterprises" make up this collection. Although the work contains imagined conversations and many factual errors, it includes some interesting sketches of Northern nurses.

Brockett, Linus Pierpont, and Mary C. Vaughn. *Women's Work in the Civil War: A Record of Heroism, Patriotism, and Patience.* Philadelphia: Zeigler, McCurdy, and Co., 1867, 799 p.

This work consists of many very brief biographies of Northern women. The many nurses include Dorothea Dix, Clara Barton, Helen Louise Gilson, Mary Bickerdyke, Mrs. William H. Holstein, Mrs. Cordelia E. P. Harvey, Katherine Prescott Wormeley, the Woolsey sisters, Annie Wittenmyer, and Annie Etheridge. Other chapters are descriptions of hospitals, such as Annapolis Hospital in the buildings of the United States Naval Academy.

Brodman, Estelle. "Memoir of Robert Fletcher." *Bulletin of the Medical Library Association* 49 (1961): 251–90.

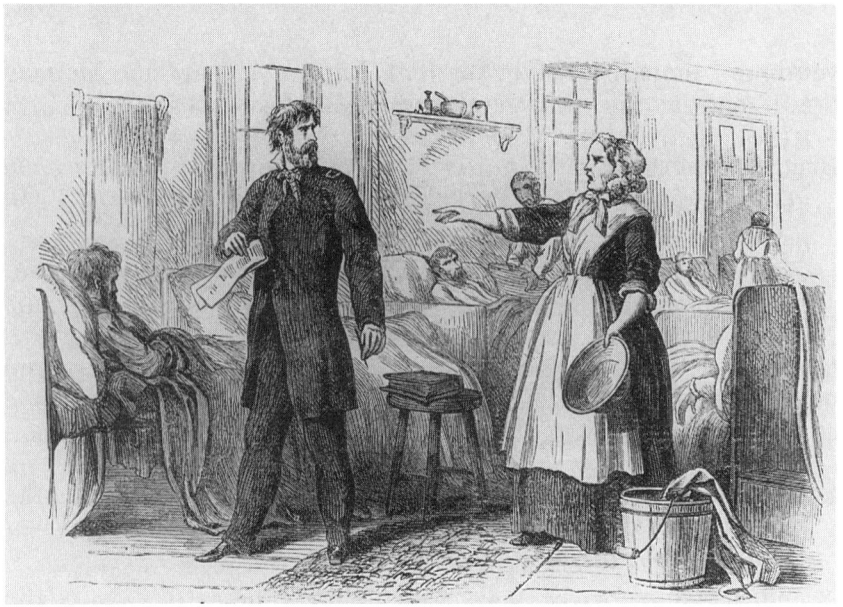

Mother Bickerdyke, the "calico cyclone," struck terror into the heart of any physician whom she thought was shirking his duty. "Here these men, any one of them worth a thousand of you, are suffered to starve and die, because you want to be off upon a drunk," she confronts the hapless surgeon in this drawing. "Pull off your shoulder straps, for you shall not stay in the army a week longer!" The surgeon went to General William T. Sherman to complain, but, when Sherman was told that Mother Bickerdyke had arranged his discharge, he told the surgeon to go home a civilian. "She ranks me." From Brockett, *Battlefield and Hospital*, 1888, pp. 296–97.

Fletcher was born in Bristol, England, in 1823 and educated in medicine there and in London. He came to the United States with his wife and child and settled in Cincinnati in 1846. He practiced medicine and then ran a drug store. When the War began, he became the surgeon of the 1st Ohio. He organized Hospital Number 1 in Nashville in two existing buildings, one of which was the Howard High School. He later supervised Hospital Number 7 (after 1863 called Number 19) and the Female Venereal Hospital for prostitutes. He was promoted in February 1863 to medical purveyor for the Army of the Cumberland. He took written examinations for various medical positions, always finishing first among examinees. Brodman has reviewed some of these examinations and found that Dr. Fletcher was extremely current in medical knowledge. He soon was providing medical supplies to the armies of Grant, Rosecrans, Sherman, and Thomas. His accounts were always accurate. Fletcher was present during the Battle of Nashville; family tradition says that his fourteen-year-old son took part in the battle. After the War, Fletcher assisted J. H. Baxter in the preparation of his work on anthropometery, then assisted J. S. Billings with the development of the *Index Medicus* and the Army Medical Library.

Brodman, Estelle, and Elizabeth B. Carrick. "American Military Medicine in the Mid-Nineteenth Century: The Experience of Alexander H. Hoff, M.D." *Bulletin of the History of Medicine* 64 (1990): 63–78.

The recent donation of the papers of Civil War surgeon Alexander H. Hoff stimulated the authors to review his life. Born in Philadelphia in 1821, Hoff graduated from the Jefferson Medical College and began practice in New York state. He was Surgeon General of New York in the 1850s and one of the first physicians to volunteer his services in 1861. Late in that year, he was sent to St. Louis, where he was placed in charge of the *D. A. January,* identified by the authors as the first hospital ship owned (not leased) by the United States Army. It was a fully fitted mobile 450-bed hospital that, during the War, transported 32,738 patients with a mortality rate of only 2.3 percent.

During the two years he served as medical director of this ship, he wrote several letters to Dr. Alden Marsh, a New York surgeon. He complained bitterly about the butchery of army surgery. Surgeon Hammond accompanied Hoff on the *D.A. January* and the two discussed the overuse of calomel by army physicians. When Hammond removed calomel from the army medical supply table (formulary), a huge outcry arose from the civilian medical community. Hoff thought that if the army contained physicians who could not use calomel properly, "better dismiss them, and get those who can." Hoff got in trouble himself when he asked a woman from the Christian Commission to desist from helping a particular soldier. She complained to the highest levels and Hoff had to explain that the soldier had to relieve himself and had asked the chief surgeon to remove the woman. "Here is one of the strong objections to female nurses," he added. In 1864, Hoff was transferred to New York harbor to supervise medical evacuation during Grant's Virginia campaign. The article includes Hoff's important postwar activities in the army.

Brooks, Stewart M. *Civil War Medicine*. Springfield, IL: Charles C. Thomas, 1966, 148 p.

This excellent but brief book covers medicine North and South. The coverage is topical, not chronological. The author seldom quotes the original literature, but gives an excellent summary of medical problems. He credits Acting Surgeon General Robert Wood with convincing Secretary of War Cameron and President Lincoln that the Army should cooperate with the United States Sanitary Commission. The author feels that Hammond and Moore were both excellent chiefs of their respective medical departments.

Bruce, Robert V. *The Launching of American Science, 1846–1876.* New York: Alfred A. Knopf, 1987, 446 p.

Bruce concludes that the Civil War retarded scientific development in the United States, both North and (especially) South. The War did raise the city of Washington, however, to the status of an American scientific center second only to Boston. Bruce relates a scientific near-miss: how the North missed the "opportunity" to develop chlorine poison gas.

Bryan, Leon S. "Blood-letting in American Medicine, 1830–1892." *Bulletin of the History of Medicine* 38 (1964): 516–29.

By studying treatment recommendations in American medical textbooks of the nineteenth century, the author notes a steady decline in blood-letting from 1830 to 1890. Opposition was never spelled out rationally; blood-letting was never debated. Its use just gradually decreased until, by 1890, blood-letting had virtually disappeared from treatment, except for diseases known to be associated with vascular congestion such as apoplexy.

Bullough, Bonnie, and Vern Bullough. "The Origins of Modern American Nursing: The Civil War Era." *Nursing Forum* 2, no. 2 (1963): 13–27.

The major message of this brief review is that the experiences of the Civil War led to the acceptance of women nurses. The article begins by describing the confusion of 1861, when one group of women concerned about military health began the United States Sanitary Commission, while another group formed around Dorothea Dix, the official "Superintendent of the United States Army Nurses." Women doctors such as Elizabeth Blackwell tried to train enthusiastic women, mostly upper-class women, into some of the rudimentary aspects of nursing. By the end of the War, doctors welcomed women nurses and the groundwork had been laid for the hospital nursing schools of the 1870s.

Burdett, Henry C. *Hospitals and Asylums of the World,* 4 vols. and portfolio. London: Churchill, 1891–93.

Volume 3 of this encyclopedic survey of hospitals and asylums includes a list of all existing civilian and military hospital in the United States. Civil War military hospitals still in use in 1890 include the Lincoln, Soldier's Home, and Harewood Hospitals in Washington, the Sedgwick Hospital of New Orleans, the Hicks Hospital in Baltimore, and the Presidio in San Francisco. The author visited Lincoln Hospital; in 1890, it held 1,240 beds, down from its Civil War maximum, including tents, of 2,575. A fence five feet high had been constructed around the entire complex sometime after the War.

Burns, Stanley B. *Early Medical Photography in America (1839–1883)*. New York: Burns Archive, 1983, various pagination.

This review of medical photography contains a chapter on Civil War photography, originally published in the *New York Journal of Medicine*. Many important photographs are reproduced, including Camp Letterman at Gettysburg and many individual operations and specimens.

Burns, Stanley B. "Focus on Photographs: Pre-Antiseptic Surgery." *Medical Heritage* 1 (1985): 465–66.

This brief survey of photography in the Civil War era points out that the surgeons wore street clothes. The article includes a photograph of an outdoor operation being performed after the Battle of Gettysburg.

C

Cantlie, Neil. *A History of the Army Medical Department,* 2 vols. Edinburgh: Churchill Livingston, 1974, 519, 448 p.

This work reviews military medical activities in Britain from the time of the New Model Army of the English Civil War to about 1900. A major focus is on the Crimean War and the "Era of Reform" immediately following. The American Civil War is not mentioned despite the fact that the British reforms were occurring about the same time as the sweeping changes in the Medical Department of the United States Army.

Carpenter, Kenneth J. *The History of Scurvy and Vitamin C*. Cambridge: Cambridge University Press, 1986, 288 p.

This overview covers scurvy from its first description to the full understanding of its prevention by vitamin C. The initial observations of James Lind concerning the prevention of scurvy on long voyages by citrus fruits were not fully accepted at the time of the Civil War.

Carrigan, Jo Ann. "Privilege, Prejudice, and the Strangers' Disease in Nineteenth-Century New Orleans." *Journal of Southern History* 36 (1970): 568–78.

In the early nineteenth century, New Orleans was notorious as a major entry point for yellow fever. The disease was especially virulent among newcomers, hence its name "the strangers' disease." This phenomenon led to a class view of yellow fever: it carried off the Irish but not the fine old families of the city. Before the Civil War, a yellow fever epidemic occurred about every other year, but, after the War, only in 1867 and 1878. During the War, many New Orleans natives hoped for a yellow fever epidemic that would sweep away the Yankees (the strangers) without damaging the local population too severely.

Carrigan, Jo Ann. "Yankees versus Yellow Jack in New Orleans, 1862–1866." *Civil War History* 9 (1963): 248–60.

The author states that some cases of yellow fever appeared in New Orleans every year from the late eighteenth century to 1860. The disorder seemed to be getting worse prior to the Civil War with severe epidemics in 1853, 1854, 1855, and 1858; these epidemics produced a total mortality in the city of almost 18,000 citizens. In 1861, the Louisiana Board of Health noted that not a single case of yellow fever had been recorded; they attributed this to the blockade. In 1862, after the Yankees took New Orleans, General Benjamin Butler developed his own theory of yellow fever prevention. He invoked a strict quarantine to keep out the "seeds" of fever that might be imported; at the same time, he cleaned up the detritus and decaying animal matter throughout the city in order to stop the spread of the disease should a case occur. Although a few cases were diagnosed in the later years of the War, no epidemic occurred. Butler attributed this to his efforts. Another Louisiana citizen had this explanation: "God was merciful and would not send to New Orleans both General Butler and yellow fever at the same time." Carrigan reviews the situation in the light of modern knowledge and claims that quarantine alone was insufficient since a few cases did occur. Luck was partly involved.

Carson, Joseph. *A History of the Medical Department of the University of Pennsylvania*. Philadelphia: Lindsay and Blakiston, 1869, 227 p.

This work barely mentions the Civil War, but does list the medical faculty of the University of Pennsylvania during the 1860s.

Cashman, Diane Cobb. *Headstrong: The Biography of Amy Morris Bradley, 1823–1904: A Life of Noble Usefulness*. Wilmington, NC: Broadfoot Publishing, 1990, 269 p.

Bradley served as a nurse in the field hospital of the 3rd Maine and at Fairfax Hospital, Alexandria, Virginia. She nursed aboard hospital transports during the Peninsula campaign. While assigned to the *Knickerbocker,* she had close daily contact with Frederick Law Olmsted, Georgy and Eliza Woolsey, Katherine Prescott Wormeley, and Helen Gilson. She served aboard the *Louisiana* with Annie Etheridge; three times the vessel traveled under flag of truce to City Point to evacuate severely wounded Union soldiers who had been prisoners. The last two years of the War, she served as an agent of the U.S. Sanitary Commission at the Rendezvous of Distribution in Alexandria, where she edited the newspaper known as *The Soldier's Journal.*

Chicago Medical Society. *History of Medicine and Surgery and Physicians and Surgeons of Chicago.* Chicago: Biographical Publishing Corporation, 1922, 928 p.

This review of Chicago medicine contains a section on nineteenth-century doctors. These biographical sketches contain Civil War medical information. Joseph S. Hildreth (1832–70), for example, was commissioned surgeon of United States Volunteers in order to put into operation an eye and ear hospital. "The old City Hospital was commandeered for that purpose. He named the establishment Des Marres Hospital after his former preceptor." Gaylord D. Beebe (1835–77) graduated from the Homeopathic Medical College of Pennsylvania in 1857 and opened a practice of homeopathic medicine in Chicago. When the War began, the local medical examining board refused to examine him. "Dr. Beebe then procured an order from President Lincoln directing the board to examine him." He passed, was commissioned, and rose within the army until he became medical director of the 14th Army Corps under General George Thomas, "by whom he was cited for especially distinguished service at Murfreesboro." Randolph Nathaniel Hall (1844–1901) was a drummer boy with the 8th Iowa, present at Shiloh and Vicksburg. After the War, he became a doctor.

Churchman, John W. "The Use of Quinine during the Civil War." *Bulletin of the Johns Hopkins Hospital* 17 (1906): 175–81.

The Union army consumed nineteen tons of quinine sulfate and nine and a half tons of sulfate of cinchona. Some was imported (the government did not pay the 45 percent import fee), but most was made from Peruvian bark by two chemical firms in Philadelphia: (1) Powers and Weightman and (2) Rosengarten and Sons.

Coburn, Mark. "The Man They Loved to Hate." *Civil War Times Illustrated* 26 (Dec. 1987): 37–43.

This article discusses the Civil War era humorist, Petroleum V. Nasby. Nasby describes the medical infirmities that prevented his enlistment in the Union army (one can imagine him talking to the examining doctor): "I'm bald-headed, and hev bin oblidged to wear a wig these 22 years. I hev dandruff in wat scanty hair still hangs around my venerable temples. I am rupchered in nine places, and am entirely enveloped with trusses. I hev verrykose veins, hev a white swellin on wun leg and a fever sore on the uther; also wun leg is shorter than tother, though I handle it so expert that nobody never noticed it."

Coco, Gregory A. *A Vast Sea of Misery: A History and Guide to the Union and Confederate Field Hospitals at Gettysburg, July 1 to November 20, 1863*. Gettysburg, PA: Thomas Publications, 1988, 208 p.

This important survey of the vast number of field hospitals in use during and after the Battle of Gettysburg includes photographs of their present appearance.

Coddington, Edward B. "Soldiers' Relief in the Seaboard States of the Southern Confederacy." *Mississippi Valley Historical Review* 37 (1950): 17–38.

This general review of the Medical Department of the Confederate States Army describes its early disorganization. Much help came from private organizations; these were never on a national basis, but were consolidated by state. In August 1861, for examples, the Richmond YMCA took responsibility for delivering packages from home to hospitalized soldiers. In another such instance, the state of North Carolina supplied North Carolina regiments in Confederate service.

Coleman, Charles H., and Paul H. Spence "The Charleston Riot, March 28, 1864." *Journal of the Illinois State Historical Society* 33 (March 1940): 7–56.

This article reviews completely the riot in Charleston, Illinois, including the killing of Surgeon Shuball York. York's son had earlier killed a Democrat or Copperhead in Mattoon, so this may have been a revenge killing. Accounts vary but probably Shuball York was shot in the back while on the second floor of the courthouse, just as the riot started outside.

Cooke, Michael A. "The Health of the Union Military in the District of Columbia, 1861–1865." *Military Affairs* 48 (1984): 194–99.

This article surveys military hospitals and the health of the Washington garrison throughout the War. By comparing statistics between the garrison troops of the city forts and the soldiers of the Army of the Potomac, the author corroborates the contemporary opinion that a moving army is healthier than a stationary one. The more common diseases among the Washington troops were diarrhea, typhoid fever, rheumatism, malaria, measles, and venereal disease. The author thinks that the worst hospital in Washington was the Cliffburn Barracks Hospital, the headquarters of the Veteran Reserve Corps. Washington was the center for broken-down horses gleaned from the overworked cavalry of the Army of the Potomac; Medical Inspector Richard H. Coolidge attributed the unhealthfulness of the nation's capital to the improper burial of dead animals. The massive influx of sick and wounded in early 1864 from the Virginia campaign required an enlargement of hospital space through the use of tents.

Courtwright, David T. "Opiate Addiction as a Consequence of the Civil War." *Civil War History* 24 (1978): 101–11.

This article analyzes the possibility that the massive use of opium and morphine during the Civil War helped to create a nationwide problem with addiction in the decades after the War. Hypodermic injection of morphine can create addiction quite readily, but not many hypodermic needles were used by army doctors (an exception being Turner's Lane Hospital for nerve injuries in Philadelphia). One can become addictied to opium also after only oral use, however. Courtwright carefully weighs the pros and the cons and concludes that Civil War opium use was a major factor in the later problem of widespread addicition.

Crandall, David L. "From Roxbury to Richmond: The Military Career of Henry P. Bowditch." *The Physiologist* 32 (1989): 88–95.

In 1887, Henry P. Bowditch was elected the first president of the American Physiological Society. As a young man twenty-five years earlier, he was a cavalry officer with the Union army. He was wounded during the Mine Run campaign in November 1863. This article includes an X ray taken in 1896 showing fragments of the ball still in place in his shoulder.

Crawford, Robert F. "The Civil War Letters of S. Rodman and Linton Smith." *Delaware History* 21 (1984): 86–116.

After studying medicine for one year at the University of Pennsylvania, Linton Smith became an assistant surgeon with the 4th

Delaware. While with the Washington garrison in January of 1863, Smith wrote his mother in Wilmington, Delaware, asking her to obtain vaccine material from the local civilian physician, William R. Bullock. Linton planned to revaccinate the men of the 4th Delaware with reliable vaccine material because of a recent smallpox scare. With his unit in the line against Petersburg in July of 1864, the surgeon of the 4th Delaware, Dickinson S. Hopkins died of typhoid fever; Smith was promoted to that position. He was busy treating the sick and wounded on the Virginia front. Two officers from his regiment were killed in action during the last week before Lee's surrender. Smith was an eyewitness to the surrender at Appomattox. After the war he ran a pharmacy in Wilmington and died at age eighty-four.

Crawley, Laura. "Civil War Hospitals around the Chickamauga Battlefield." *Journal of the Medical Association of Georgia* 78 (1989): 279–81.

This brief article summarizes the Confederate medical care at the Battle of Chickamauga.

Crawley, Laura. *Civil War Medicine at the Chickamauga Battlefield.* Rossville, GA: privately printed, 1986, 19 p.

This excellent account of medical care at the Battle of Chickamauga includes locations of field hospitals.

Cullan, Joseph P. "Chimborazo Hospital: That Charnal House of Living Sufferers." *Civil War Times Illustrated* 29 (January 1981): 36–42.

The author (whose name is spelled Cullen on the title page but Cullan in the index) argues that a study of the original Chimborago records provides a more somber analysis of hospital conditions than that of the rosy descriptions written long after the War. After the battles near Richmond in the summer of 1862, the existing buildings became overcrowded and filthy. Dr. McCaw refused to accept additional wounded, but the ambulance drivers just dumped them in the streets of the hospital compound. They were placed on the floors of the buildings, in spaces between beds, until about 3,500 patients were present. The author wishes to demolish two myths: Southern women volunteered for hospital work in droves (actually Chimborazo never filled its allotment of matrons) and Chimborazo had a mortality rate less than 10 percent. By counting graves in the Oakwood Cemetery, the author claims that at least 20 percent of the patients admitted to Chimborazo died.

Culpepper, Marilyn Mayer, and Pauline Gordon Adams. "Nursing in the Civil War." *American Journal of Nursing* 88 (1988): 981–84.

This brief article reviews the activities of many of the female volunteers, matrons, and Sanitary Commission representatives. Male nurses are not mentioned.

Cunningham, Horace H. "The Confederate Medical Officer in the Field." *New York Academy of Medicine Bulletin* 34 (1958): 461–88.

This excellent article describes the duties of the regimental medical officers. Cunningham begins by describing the chain of command, including the separation of general hospitals from control of the medical directors of armies by an order of 12 March 1863. He lists the efforts of medical officers, only partially successful, to maintain camp cleanliness. He describes the daily medical routine, including sick call. The activities of the regimental medical officer in battle makes up a large part of this essay. These activities included the preparations for battle, directing the "infirmary corps" of about thirty noncombatants to remove the wounded, and initial treatment at the field infirmary (aid station). Some surgery took place there. The author then considers the problems of evacuation, including ambulance wagons. These wagons and the animals to draw them were always in short supply; the animals were often broken down (probably most were rejects from the cavalry). Rail transportation was the final step to the general hospital system.

Efforts to coordinate the Medical, Commissary, and Quartermaster departments were largely unsuccessful. Despite Surgeon General Moore's many efforts, no plan of coordination was ever adopted. The final section considers the treatment of captured Union wounded soldiers and doctors; despite several examples of inhumanity, both the South and the North generally conducted themselves so well that the medical example helped "the restoration of an harmonious Union" after the War. This essay seems to be more scholarly in tone and flow than the author's book published the same year.

Cunningham, Horace H. *Doctors in Gray: The Confederate Medical Service*. Baton Rouge: Louisiana State University Press, 1958, 339 p.

This is the standard book on Confederate medicine. The bibliographic essay gives the location of the manuscript papers of many leading Confederate doctors. Many references to published articles, however, are incorrect.

Cunningham, Horace H. *Field Medical Services at the Battles of Manassas (Bull Run)*. Athens: University of Georgia Press, 1968, 116 p.

The author discusses in detail both Union and Confederate medical care at both battles at Bull Run. The medical services of both combatants were disorganized at First Manassas. During the following year, the North improved its medical care much more than the South. Northern military medical care was considerably superior to Southern medical efforts at Second Manassas.

D

Dammann, Gordon. *Pictorial Encyclopedia of Civil War Medical Instruments and Equipment,* 2 vols. Missoula, MT: Pictorial Histories Publishing Company, vol. 1:1983, 100 p. and vol. 2:1988, 96 p.

Most medical procedures and artefacts are illustrated, including uniforms, surgical instruments, and medical kits as well as hospitals and ambulances.

Dannett, Sylvia G. L. "Lincoln's Ladies in White." *New York State Journal of Medicine* 61 (1961): 1944–52.

This essay reviews the role of Northern women in the War. It includes the founding of the United States Sanitary Commission, the use of women in hospitals and on hospital transports, and the difficulty women had after the War in obtaining government pensions for war service. The author thinks that Dorothea Dix was more of a barrier than a stimulation to the use of women nurses.

Davenport, Horace W. "Such Is Military: Dr. George Martin Trowbridge's Letters from Sherman's Army, 1863–1865." *New York Academy of Medicine Bulletin* 63 (1987): 844–82.

Trowbridge became assistant surgeon with the 19th Michigan after graduating from the medical faculty of the University of Michigan in 1862. One of his duties was "quinine call," when he personally supervised the administration of quinine, mixed in whiskey, to every soldier in the regiment. His greatest dislike was performing a difficult operation and then having the patient transferred to a hospital in the rear; he lost the follow-up necessary for professional growth, but "such is military" (his comment on every aspect of military medicine that he did not like). He treated a rebel "bushwhacker" who was paraplegic after being shot in the back. The patient complained of cold feet, and his friends put heated rocks near his feet. Unfortunately he could not feel heat because of spinal cord dysfunction; his feet were severely burned and he lost several toes.

At the start of the Georgia campaign, Trowbridge noted that the poor diet of the troops might bring on scurvy. "Unless we get vegetables, there will be trouble with scurvy among us," he wrote to his wife on 19 May 1864. He noted no scurvy among rebel prisoners. Scurvy remained a problem until berries began to appear on the bushes. In Atlanta, he set up the 2nd Division Hospital, 14th Army Corps, in the old Medical College Hospital buildings. He was proud that no erysipelas or gangrene occurred in this hospital, although both had bothered the rebels when they had used the same building. He knew something big was up when he received orders to evacuate all the sick and wounded to Chattanooga. He then went with Sherman's army through Georgia, South Carolina, and North Carolina. He complained that so much of South Carolina was burning that the smoke continually reddened his eyes.

Davis, Ruth W. "Behind the Battle of Gettysburg American Nursing Is Born." *Pennsylvania Heritage* 13 (Fall 1987): 10–15.

The author argues that it took the first two years of the War "for physicians and military authorities to decide that they desperately needed the help of [female] nurses to tend to the victims of war." The Battle of Gettysburg proved the value of female volunteer nurses. "When women were accepted, working alongside the surgeons at Gettysburg, nursing was forged," concludes the author.

Dedmond, Francis B. "Here among Soldiers in Hospital: An Unpublished Letter from Walt Whitman to Lucia Jane Russell Briggs." *New England Quarterly* 59 (1988): 544–48.

The author relates how Whitman obtained funds to buy items for wounded soldiers (and presumably to maintain himself) by writing to New England acquaintances. Some of the members of the transcendental school would not send him any money because of what Dedmond calls "New England prudery." A more blunt contemporary wrote Whitman that his trouble was "that you are not ashamed of your reproductive organs." The essay includes a short letter of thanks from Whitman to a Mrs. Briggs who donated $75. On 26 April 1864, Whitman noted that the number of sick are "becoming alarmingly greater," suffering from "diarrhea, rheumatism, and the old camp fevers." The Army of the Potomac was emptying its division and brigade hospitals in preparation for the Wilderness campaign.

Donald, W. J. "Alabama Confederate Hospitals." *Alabama Review* 15 (1962): 271–81; 16 (1963): 64–78.

This article lists every Confederate hospital in Alabama. Many were started by private individuals or organizations and only later taken over by the Confederate government. The first was the Soldier's Home of Montgomery, started by the Ladies Aid Society on 14 June 1861. Surgeon R. L. Brodie, medical director of the Division of the West, inspected Alabama hospitals, dating his report 26 December 1864. The capacity and present census of each hospital is given. All hospitals were "well supplied with medicines with the exception of quinine, of which there is a scarcity." One hospital, the former United States Naval Hospital of Mobile, under the command of Surgeon L. L. Nidelet, had been closed because of hospital gangrene. Alabama produced fifty-eight doctors for the Confederate Army and Navy; of these fifty-six had medical degrees. The University of Pennyslvania had awarded twenty-one of these M.D. degrees and Jefferson Medical College of Philadelphia twelve.

Drayton, Evelyn S. "William Alexander Hammond, 1828–1900." *Military Surgeon* 109 (1951): 559–65.

This brief survey of Hammond's life emphasizes his military career.

Duffy, John. *The Rudolph Matas History of Medicine in Louisiana,* 2 vols. Baton Rouge: Louisiana State University Press, 1962, 599 p., 522 p.

Medical experiences during the Civil War in Louisiana are related in a large section at the beginning of volume 2. Both Confederate and Union medicine are described. New Orleans became a major center for Federal Hospitals. Union soldiers admitted to the Charity Hospital had their daily charges paid by the United States government.

Duffy, John. *Sword of Pestilence: The New Orleans Yellow Fever Epidemic of 1853.* Baton Rouge: Louisiana State University Press, 1966, 191 p.

The author thinks that the 1853 yellow fever outbreak was the single greatest epidemic to ever attack an American city. The disaster stimulated public health thinking in the South, but did not lead to the development of quarantine. In fact, the quarantine station established at the mouth of the Mississippi was closed even before the epidemic had quite spent itself.

Duffy, John. "Yellow Fever in the Continental United States during the Nineteenth Century." *New York Academy of Medicine Bulletin* 44 (1968): 687–701.

In the eighteenth century, yellow fever epidemics had been just as frequent in northern as in southern port cities of the United States. The last northern outbreak was in 1822 in New York, although cases did appear thereafter at port quarantine stations. Duffy attributes the success to quarantine and isolation measures. But in the southeastern United States, the disease continued to break out; the last epidemic was in New Orleans in 1905. During the Civil War, the blockade and the disruption of trade "undoubtedly played a role in keeping yellow fever to a minimum." The chief Civil War epidemics occurred in Charleston, Wilmington, New Bern, Pensacola, Key West, and Galveston.

Duffy, John. *The Healers: A History of American Medicine.* Urbana: University of Illinois Press, 1979, 385 p.

This survey of American medicine includes a chapter on the Civil War, but it is especially valuable in its description of American medicine as it existed just before the War.

Duffy, John. "The Impact of Malaria on the South." In *Disease and Distinctiveness in the American South,* edited by Todd L. Savitt and James Harvey Young, 29–54. Knoxville: University of Tennessee Press, 1988.

After reviewing the serious medical problem of malaria during the Civil War, Duffy concludes that "inasmuch as malaria plagued troops on both sides, it is doubtful that it had any major impact upon the outcome of the War. Although the disease was more likely to take a serious form with northern troops, they were better fed, clothed, and housed, which helped them to resist disease, and their superior numbers more than compensated for any losses incurred from malaria."

Duncan, Louis C. "The Strange Case of Surgeon-General Hammond." *Military Surgeon* 64 (1929): 98–110, 252–62.

This detailed review of Hammond's court-martial covers preliminaries, charges, and subsequent developments. The author, a leading military physician and historian, concludes that Hammond's "services to the Republic were great enough to far outweigh any trifling foibles of character."

Duncan, Louis C. *The Medical Department of the United States*

Army in the Civil War [offprints]. Washington, DC: 1910. Reprint. Gaithersburg, MD: Butternut Press, 1985, 407 p.

A United States Army physician wrote this major work on the Medical Department of the Union Army, with emphasis on the east. A comparison of illness and death rates in different wars is appended. The work was originally published as a series of articles in the *Military Surgeon*. In fact, the first edition of the book merely bound offprints of these articles together.

Dunkelman, Mark, and Michael Winey. "A Southern Nurse and a Northern Patient." *Civil War Times Illustrated* 26 (February 1988): 24–27.

A woman named Fannie Jackson was living in north Georgia, her husband away with Confederate forces, when Sherman's army passed by. A wounded Northern soldier was boarded at her house. He died from his ankle wound when a second amputation was required after the war. Although Mrs. Jackson was loyal to the South, she had three children to support and took a job as nurse in a Union army hospital in Chattanooga.

Durham, Walter T. *Nashville: The Occupied City.* Nashville: Tennessee Historical Society, 1985, 307 p.

This discussion of Nashville during 1861 and 1862 gives the location of all Confederate hospitals and, after the occupation, all Federal hospitals.

E

Epler, Percy H. *The Life of Clara Barton.* New York: Macmillan, 1926, 438 p.

This laudatory biography frequently quotes extensively from contemporary letters by Clara Barton and others. About a third of the book contains her experiences as a volunteer nurse during the Civil War; she received the apellation of the "angel of the battlefield." She helped evacuate the wounded from Second Manassas, Antietam, and Fredericksburg. She was at Hilton Head in 1863, treating the wounded from the battles around Charleston, including the attack upon Fort Wagner glorified in the film *Glory.* She nursed in the support hospitals during the final Virginia campaign of 1864–65.

Ernst, Kathleen. "An Angel from Wisconsin." *Civil War Times Illustrated* 28 (March 1989): 20–25.

This article briefly reviews the Civil War career of Cordelia Harvey, widow of the Wisconsin governor. She visited sick and wounded Wisconsin soldiers, especially in St. Louis hospitals and became determined that they would recuperate faster in a hospital in Wisconsin. After much effort, she finally obtained permission to construct such a hospital. The author accepts contemporary opinions about the effect on health: "Harvey quickly realized many of the men would benefit from time spent in the cool air of their home state."

Eyler, John M. *Victorian Social Medicine: The Ideas and Methods of William Farr.* Baltimore: Johns Hopkins University Press, 1979, 262 p.

This book concerns the life and work of Englishman William Farr, whose nosologic methods were used by both the Union and the Confederate Army Medical Bureaus. Farr's studies of illness during the Crimean War and in the peacetime British Army were a stimulus for the formation of the American sanitary commissions and influenced efforts at sanitation and disease prevention.

F

Faust, Drew Gilpin. "Altars of Sacrifice: Confederate Women and the Narratives of War." *Journal of American History* 76 (1990): 1200–28.

This work is written to counter the "celebratory myth" that all Southern women supported the War. The author states that recent scholarship has emphasized the deterioration of Confederate morale, especially on the home front, as a factor to explain Southern defeat. Most of this scholarship has emphasized class conflict; the present work emphasizes gender. A typical sentence is: "War has been a preeminently gendering activity, casting thought about sex differences into sharp relief as it has both underlined and realigned gender boundaries." The article does not mention the work of women in Confederate hospitals. [The reviewer cannot help but think that some professional historians have lost contact with those who want to understand the past.]

Fishbein, Morris. *A History of the American Medical Association, 1847 to 1947.* Philadelphia: W. B. Saunders, 1947, 1226 p.

This encyclopedic history of the American Medical Association provides a short summary of each national meeting including those of the Civil War era. An appendix summarizes the lives of all AMA presidents, including their War service. A large number in the postwar era were veterans of the Confederate army: W. O. Baldwin, 1869, D. W. Yandell (Medical Director, Department of the West under Albert Sydney Johnston), 1872, W. K. Bowling, 1875, T. C. Richardson, 1878, H. F. Campbell (who had been in charge of the Georgia section of Chimborazo Hospital, Richmond), 1885, A. Y. P. Garnett (personal physician of Jefferson Davis), 1888, and John A. Wyeth (a private during the War), 1902.

Foltz, Charles S. *Surgeon of the Seas: The Adventurous Life of Surgeon General Jonathan M. Foltz in the Days of Wooden Ships.* Indianapolis, IN: Bobbs-Merrill, 1931, 351 p.

J. M. Foltz was a surgeon on Farragut's flagship, the U.S.S. *Hartford,* when the fleet captured New Orleans and bombarded Grand Gulf, Mississippi. He served on the Mississippi River and was present during the siege of Vicksburg. From late in 1863 to the end of the war, he served with the Naval Medical Examining Board in Philadelphia. He was later surgeon general of the Navy. This book includes many direct quotations from his diary, but contains little of direct medical interest.

Franke, Norman H. "Official and Industrial Aspects of Pharmacy in the Confederacy." *Georgia Historical Quarterly* 37 (1953): 175–87.

This article reviews the Medical Bureau of the Confederate States Army with excellent photographs of Moore and McGuire. It quotes extensively from Moore's circulars. Franke examines pharmacy laboratories in the Confederacy with most emphasis on the Mohr lab in Mobile.

Franke, Norman H. "Pharmaceutical Conditions and Drug Supply in the Confederacy." *Georgia Historical Quarterly* 37 (1953): 287–98.

This article examines efforts to bring drugs through the blockade. Mohr was afraid that the smugglers accidently mixed up quinine sulfate and morphine sulfate.

Franke, Norman H. "Pharmacy and Pharmacists in the Confederacy." *Georgia Historical Quarterly* 38 (1954): 11–28.

The third and final section of Franke's review of Confederacy pharmaceutical efforts concerns efforts to substitute indigenous substances for imported ones. A table lists inactive substitutes for quinine, calomel, and other drugs. Attempts to obtain quinine substitutes centered upon tree bark bitter to the taste.

Fredrickson, George M. *The Inner Civil War: Northern Intellectuals and the Crisis of the Union.* New York: Harper and Row, 1965, 277 p.

The Civil War caused Northern intellectuals to reassess the basis of their beliefs. Different people had different responses to the War and its carnage. The two responses of medical interest were the effort of humanitarian individuals to relieve suffering, as exemplified by volunteer nurses, and the formation of the United States Sanitary Commission by members of the conservative elite. The major contribution of the Commission was to show "the need for an expert to act as intermediary between irrational popular benevolence and the suffering to be relieved."

Freemon, Frank R. "The Health of the American Slave Examined by Means of Union Army Medical Statistics." *Journal of the National Medical Association* 77 (1985): 49–52.

The author masterfully compares the health of black and white Union soldiers. He probably goes beyond the evidence, however, when he tries to use this information to determine the health of slaves before they became soldiers.

Freemon, Frank R. "Administration of the Medical Department of the Confederate States Army, 1861 to 1865." *Southern Medical Journal* 80 (1987): 630–37.

This article is an incredibly brilliant analysis and exposition of the Confederate Medical Bureau in Richmond.

Freemon, Frank R. "Lincoln Finds a Surgeon General: William A. Hammond and the Transformation of the Union Army Medical Bureau." *Civil War History* 33 (1987): 5–21.

This essay provides a scintillating narrative of Hammond's Civil War career. The author analyzes the role of Hammond in the successes and failures of the Union Medical Department.

Freemon, Frank R. "The Siege of Vicksburg, 1863: How Medicine Affected the Outcome." *New York Academy of Medicine Bulletin* 67 (1991): 429–38.

This essay is a brilliant review of published and manuscript medical statistics concerning the siege at Vicksburg.

Fye, W. Bruce. "S. Weir Mitchell, Philadelphia's Lost Physiologist." *Bulletin of the History of Medicine* 57 (1983): 188–202.

Silas Weir Mitchell was a leading candidate for the chair of physiology at the University of Pennsylvania in 1863. Despite support from such leading scientists as Joseph Henry and Louis Agassiz, he was not chosen. The author thinks that this defeat helped to produce a shift in his intellectual interests from animal research to a study of nervous system disorders that he was then encountering as a contract surgeon. After the War, the city had another chance to prevent Mitchell from becoming "Philadelphia's lost physiologist." But in 1868, Mitchell was also defeated for the chair of physiology at Jefferson Medical College. He went on to a major career in neurology and was a founding member in 1887 of the American Physiological Society.

G

Garrison, Fielding H. *John Shaw Billings: A Memoir.* New York: Putnam's, 1915, 432 p.

This biography of Billings, based largely on his letters, contains a chapter on his activities during the War. Billings was the medical director of Georgetown and Cliffburne Hospitals and was present at the battles of Chancellorsville and Gettysburg.

Garrison, Fielding H. "The Statistical Lessons of the Crimean War." *Military Surgeon* 41 (1917): 457–73.

This article contains extensive mortality and illness statistics from the Crimean War. At the time Garrison wrote, the Crimean War held two statistical records: the Russians had the greatest losses in battle (killed in action) per 1,000 troops engaged and the French had the highest number of deaths due to sickness per 1,000 troops engaged.

Garrison, Fielding H. *Notes on the History of Military Medicine.* Washington, DC: Government Printing Office, 1922, 206 p.

This major work is based upon the author's articles in *Military Surgeon.* The author examines each war in Europe and in America including available health statistics. The review of the American Civil War emphasizes the development of the Letterman system.

Gay, Evelyn W. *The Medical Profession in Georgia.* Fulton, MO: Ovid Bell Press, 1983, 447 p.

This book contains one chapter on Georgia doctors in the Civil War. Many interesting people are described, such as Paul F. Eve, who was present after the Battle of Solferino. He was surgeon

176

general of the state of Tennessee and surgeon-in-charge of Gate City Hospital, Atlanta. The most interesting anecdote concerns how Dr. Noel D'Alvigny saved the Atlanta Medical College building from being destroyed by Sherman's troops. The lower level of the building was filled with straw, but when Union officers arrived to ignite it on 14 November 1864, D'Alvigny informed them that he had been unable to evacuate the paralyzed patients on the second floor. A hurried inspection revealed a number of bedridden individuals groaning in agony. The Union officers gave D'Alvigny a day to evacuate these patients, who were actually nurses and able-bodied soldiers shamming illness. When the day was up, Sherman's troops had all left Atlanta, just as D'Alvigny had suspected they would, and the Atlanta Medical College was saved.

Gaston, Kay Baker. "A World Overturned: The Civil War Experience of Dr. William A. Cheatham and his Family." *Tennessee Historical Quarterly* 50 (1991): 3–16.

Dr. William A. Cheatham, a cousin of General Benjamin F. Cheatham of the Army of Tennessee, graduated from the University of Pennsylvania Medical School in 1843. He helped to develop the first mental hospital in Tennessee and was appointed its director in 1852. For the next ten years, he gained national stature for his treatment of mental illness. During the first year of the War, as opposing armies marched along the Murfreesboro Road in front of the Tennessee Hospital for the Insane, his main concern was to obtain supplies for the 300 inmates, "more than two thirds of which are bereft of reason." He often was unable to pay the hospital workers because of lack of funds. In 1862, the new military governor, Andrew Johnson, replaced Cheatham for political reasons. One of the great social events in the short life of the Confederacy was the marriage of Cheatham's wife's sister to John Hunt Morgan.

Gibson, John M. *Soldier in White: The Life of General George Miller Sternberg*. Durham, NC: Duke University Press, 1958, 277 p.

A chapter in Sternberg's biography covers his Civil War service with emphasis upon his capture at First Manassas. Sternberg also served in the Peninsula campaign and in the Trans-Mississippi theater.

Gillett, Mary C. "A Tale of Two Surgeons." *Medical Heritage* 1 (1985): 404–13.

An interesting comparison of the careers of Joseph C. Woodward and George M. Sternberg, this article includes their test scores on their army entrance examinations. Woodward had a brilliant Civil War career, but had difficulty accepting the germ theory of disease.

Gillett, Mary C. *The Army Medical Department, 1818–1865*. Washington, DC: Government Printing Office, 1987, 371 p.

This official history of United States Army medicine gives a great deal of attention to army doctors in the west in the antebellum years. Civil War medicine is covered chronologically from the Northern point of view. This excellent narrative may replace Adams' *Doctors in Blue* as the standard history of Union army medicine.

Goff, Richard D. *Confederate Supply*. Durham, NC: Duke University Press, 1969, 275 p.

This book reviews the overwhelming difficulties of the Confederate States Army in obtaining and distributing supplies. The Surgeon General's Office in 1863 had twenty-one clerks and directed seven drug manufactures and four alcohol distilleries, but still obtained most of its supplies by capture and by importation through the blockade.

Gould, Benjamin A. *Investigation in the Military and Anthropological Statistics of American Soldiers*. New York: Hurd and Houghton, 1869, 655 p.

This official publication of the United States Sanitary Commission contains a wealth of statistical information about the Union soldier, such as average height, weight, and other measurements. The last section contains a monthly statement of the total Union army effectives, wounded, sick, and other categories, but nothing on specific diseases.

Gow, June I. "Theory and Practice in Confederate Military Administration." *Military Affairs* 39 (1975): 119–23.

This article is mainly about Samuel Cooper, who at age sixty-three, became adjutant and inspector general of the Confederate States Army; he had been adjutant general of the United States Army from 1852 until 1861. Cooper saw his role mainly as an administrator to file reports and route correspondence, not as a link in the military chain of command. The article contains some information on the status of the surgeon general within the Confederate military bureaucracy; he reported to the secretary of war.

Griffith, Lucille "Mrs. Juliet Opie Hopkins and Alabama Military Hospitals." *Alabama Review* 6 (1953): 99–120.

Mrs. Hopkins was the wife of a former United States Senator who became the chief justice of the Alabama Supreme Court during the War. She helped to organize and run the "Alabama Hospital," which the Confederacy considered one division of the Chimborazo Hospital, but which she considered a state institution. She took funds raised by such organizations as the Ladies Aid Association of Montgomery to purchase food and other items needed by the wounded and sick soldiers in the Alabama Hospital in Richmond. Mrs. Hopkins was herself wounded (apparently slightly) at the Battle of Seven Pines while aiding the evacuation of wounded soldiers.

Gurdjian, E. Stephen. "The Treatment of Penetrating Wounds of the Brain Sustained in Warfare: A Historical Review." *Journal of Neurosurgery* 39 (1974): 157–67.

This excellent historical review emphasizes penetrating missle wounds of the brain. The American Civil War is not specifically mentioned.

Hall, Courtney R. "Confederate Medicine." *Medical Life* 42 (1935): 443–508.

This long article took up an entire issue of *Medical Life.* An introduction discusses how the War began with emphasis on the perfidy of the North. A chapter on medical organization concludes that Moore was the ideal surgeon general: studious, efficient, and forceful. Chapters on hospitals and on regimental surgeons are excellent. A final chapter reviews the effect of the war upon ordinary soldiers, doctors, and women. As a major source, Hall uses the *Dictionary of American Biography.*

Hall, Courtney R. "The Rise of Professional Surgery in the United States, 1800–1865." *Bulletin of the History of Medicine* 26 (1952): 231–62.

This review of American surgery contains a section on the major influence of the Civil War.

Hall, Courtney R. "The Lessons of the War Between the States." *International Record of Medicine* 171 (1958): 408–30.

This article reviews the medical efforts of both the North and the South. The author thinks that the Confederate medical effort was "valiant and commendable," but the problems were so great that "no medical department or staff could have made the lot of the Confederate soldier much better." In weighing the medical pluses and minuses, Hall finds the War a mixed blessing. A huge medical and surgical experience was gathered, probably improving the civilian practices of the former military doctors. The author thinks that "medical education underwent some deterioration" after the War, partly due to the destruction of Southern medical schools and the movement into the unsettled West. Women nurses in the Civil War set the pattern for a nursing profession for women. The author is most ambivalent about the effect of the War upon civilian public health. In the first place, "the coming of the war put an end to a promising public health movement." But in 1869, Massachusetts established the first state board of health and nineteen other states had followed this lead within a decade. The American Public Health Association was formed in 1872 by a number of men active in the Medical Department and in the Sanitary Commission.

Haller, John S. "Civil War Anthropometry: The Making of a Racial Ideology." *Civil War History* 16 (1970): 309–24.

Extensive measurements of soldiers were made by the Provost-Marshal-General Bureau (in charge of the draft) and by the United States Sanitary Commission. After the War, these physical measurements (anthropometry), amplified by autopsy measures, particularly brain weights, were reanalyzed by race. The author concludes that "nearly all subsequent late-nineteenth-century institutionalized attitudes of racial inferiority focussed upon the war anthropometry as the basis of their belief." He notes the irony that the War that ended race slavery contributed to the scientific theory of racial inferiority.

Haller, John S., Jr. *American Medicine in Transition, 1840–1910.* Urbana: University of Illinois Press, 1981, 457 p.

This survey contains no direct coverage of the Civil War, but gives a good picture of medical sects in the era. The book discusses the Hammond calomel controversy as an attempt to make therapeutics more scientific.

Hanchette, William. "An Illinois Physician and the Civil War Draft, 1864–1865: Letters of Dr. Joshua Nichols Speed." *Journal of the Illinois State Historical Society* 59 (1966): 143–60.

This article concerns the medical examination of draftees in the Ninth Congressional District of Illinois, a district centered on Mt. Sterling. The National Conscription Act of 3 March 1863 required a quota of soldiers from each Congressional District. When the quota was not met by volunteers, draftees were chosen by lot. They were examined by Dr. Roland M. Worthington and his assistant, Dr. Joshua Nichols Speed. Speed was a civilian doctor who lived in nearby Rushville and walked to Mt. Sterling each Monday morning and back every Friday night. In letters home, he gives no details of his examination methods, only that some people he examined passed and some did not. He noted that draftees hoped they would fail the examination while substitutes hired by draftees to take their place hoped that they would pass so they could receive their money.

Harris, Brayton, and Kathleen Kelley. "Invisible Enemies." *Civil War: The Magazine of the Civil War Society* (May–June 1991): 26–29.

The invisible enemies of the Civil War soldier were infected wounds, diseases, poor nutrition, and poor sanitation. The physicians of the era "did the best they could."

Harris, Brayton, and Kathleen Kelley. "Myths and Miracles: Medicine in the Civil War." *Civil War: The Magazine of the Civil War Society* 9 (May–June 1991): 18–22.

This brief review of the medical problems at the start of the Civil War concludes that "a compelling case can be made that battles were lost—or never joined—because of armies debilitated by disease."

Harrison, Gordon. *Mosquitoes, Malaria and Man: A History of the Hostilities Since 1880.* New York: E. P. Dutton, 1978, 314 p.

This book is an excellent description of the discovery of the role of the mosquito in the life cycle of the malaria parasite. Only one short chapter discusses malaria prior to this discovery.

Hartzler, Daniel D. *Medical Doctors of Maryland in the C.S.A.* Gaithersburg, MD: Olde Soldier Books, 1979, 98 p.

This book contains brief biographies of the 208 Maryland doctors who joined the Confederate States Army or Navy.

Hattaway, Herman, and Archer Jones. *How the North Won: A Military History of the Civil War.* Urbana: University of Illinois Press, 1983, 762 p.

This detailed military history of the Civil War argues that the North won because of superior utilization of its greater resources. The authors point to the Vietnam War to reject the thesis that the North's resources alone guaranteed victory. They conclude that "the South, more prone to individualism, less institutionalized, and a great deal behind the North in adoption of modern business and managerial techniques generally, could not match its adversary in effective organization." Medicine is not mentioned but could provide an example of this thesis.

Hawk, Alan. "Transportation of the Wounded: The Models of the Armed Forces Medical Museum." *Caduceus: A Museum Quarterly for the Health Sciences* 3 (Winter 1987): 1–25.

The author examines several models in the collection of the Armed Forces Medical Museum at the Armed Forces Institute of Pathology in Washington. Of Civil War interest are models of two four-wheeled ambulances: the Wheeler that could carry two stretchers or ten men seated and the Rucker that could carry four stretchers in two tiers. Models are also shown of a hospital railroad car of the Army of the Cumberland and two hospital ships. The *D. A. January,* used on the Western rivers, was a floating hospital with facilities for the performance of surgery. The *J. K. Barnes,* designed for transportation of sick and wounded up the coast, carried a total of 3,655 patients during the War; only twenty-five of these died. The *Barnes* had no operative suite since surgery could not be performed on a pitching ship in the Atlantic.

Hay, James. "Surgeons of the Confederacy: William Hay." *Confederate Veteran* 34 (1926): 9.

The author briefly describes the activities of his father, who was surgeon of the 33rd Virginia. He was later surgeon-in-charge of Staunton Hospital, but died of pneumonia on 4 June 1864.

Heck, Albert F. "William Alexander Hammond: 1828–1900." *Journal of the American Medical Association* 183 (1963): 466–68.

This brief review of Hammond's life emphasizes his accomplishments in civilian medicine following his military career.

Heitman, Francis B. *Historical Register and Dictionary of the United States Army from its Organization, September 29, 1989 to March 2, 1903,* 2 vols. Washington, DC: Government Printing Office, 1903. Reprint. Urbana: University of Illinois Press, 1965.

The first volume lists all medical officers who resigned commissions in the United States Army in order to join the Confederate States Army. The second volume contains an alphabetical listing of army officers that includes medical officers serving with the regular (but not volunteer) Union army.

Henle, Ellen Langenheim. "Clara Barton, Soldier or Pacifist?" *Civil War History* 24 (1978): 152–60.

The author reviews Clara Barton's accomplishments in providing succor to the sick and wounded during the Civil War. By quoting her letters, the author concludes that Barton would rather have been a combat soldier than a nurse.

Henry, Frederick P. *Standard History of the Medical Profession of Philadelphia*. Chicago: Goodspeed Brothers, 1897, 544 p.

The first military hospital in Philadelphia was the Christian Street Hospital, opened with one patient on 6 May 1861 in a commissioner's hall called Moyamensing Hall. Late in 1861, Philadelphia was chosen to be a hospital site second only to Washington in importance. The old railway depot at Broad and Cherry Streets was selected as chief distribution hospital and refurbished with 580 beds on three floors. The hospital at 16th and Filbert had been an arsenal and was later made famous as the scene of Mitchell's *In War Time*. Construction was begun on 1 May 1862 and completed on 6 June of the West Philadelphia or Satterlee Hospital, later enlarged to 3,500 beds. A city survey in December 1864 showed 14,508 hospital beds in fifteen military hospitals, occupied at that time by 8,638 patients. The book contains a huge list of Philadelphia physicians serving with the Union army.

Henry, Robert S. *The Armed Forces Institute of Pathology: Its First Century, 1862–1962*. Washington, DC: Government Printing Office, 1964, 422 p.

This history contains a great deal of information about the founding and earliest period of the Armed Forces Institute of Pathology.

Hill, Jim Dan. *The Civil War Sketchbook of Charles Ellery Stedman, Surgeon, United States Navy*. San Rafael, CA: Presidio Press, 1976, 218 p.

The heart of this book is a series of drawings by Surgeon Stedman, United States Navy. During 1862, he served on board the sailing ship U.S.S. *Huron,* assigned to the South Atlantic Squadron. He was present at the capture of the ports of eastern Florida, but most of the year was spent in chasing blockade runners. The next year he was aboard the ironclad monitor U.S.S. *Nahant,* bombarding forts in Charleston harbor. In 1864, he was again aboard a sailing ship, the U.S.S. *Circassian,* on cruises between Boston and the Gulf of Mexico. The written material by Hill gives a superb picture of the life of a doctor a sea. This book is essential for anyone interested in Civil War naval medicine.

Hillman, Bruce Joel. "Their Floating Palace: The Union's Hospital Boat *Red Rover*." *Civil War Times Illustrated* 24 (October 1985): 20–25.

The *Red Rover* was built at Cape Girardeau, Missouri, in 1859 for civilian trade. In November of 1861, she was purchased by the Confederate government and used as a barracks ship at Island Number 10. During the Union naval attack on that bastion, the C.S.S. *Red Rover* was struck by a shell that went all the way through her. She was captured and outfitted in St. Louis for use by the United States Navy as a hospital vessel. Such a vessel was needed: sick and wounded sailors remained aboard their vessels, often in makeshift tents on deck. But when the ship was cleared for action, these sick and wounded were unceremoniously hustled below in a dangerous manner. In June of 1862, sick and wounded from around the river fleet were transferred to the new U.S.S. *Red Rover*. The captain of the vessel was George D. Wise and the chief doctor was George H. Bixby of Boston. Nursing was supplied by the Sisters of the Holy Cross.

Hodges, Robert E., James Hood, John E. Canham, Howerde E. Sauberlich, and Eugene M. Baker. "Clinical Manifestations of Ascorbic Acid Deficiency in Man." *American Journal of Clinical Nutrition* 24 (1977): 432–43.

This study is from the famous Iowa City nutrition group. Five volunteer prison inmates were placed on a diet totally free of vitamin C. About ninety days later, they developed petechial hemorrhages and within a few days days full-blown clinical scurvy: ecchymoses, subconjunctival hemorrhages, puffy gums, hair loss, painful joints with effusions, edema, and difficulty breathing. They did not go through a stage of lassitude and weariness, as with naturally occurring scurvy (the "scorbutic taint") possibly because they went directly from a diet high in vitamin C to one with vitamin C totally absent.

Hoff, John Van R. "Memoir of Alexander Henry Hoff." *Military Surgeon* 31 (1912): 47–51.

The author writes a biography of his father. He was born in Philadelphia and graduated from Jefferson Medical School in 1843, where his preceptor was J. K. Mitchell, the father of Silas Weir Mitchell. In 1861, he became surgeon of the 3rd New York; a lantern was shot out of his hand at Big Bethel, the first battle of the War. In August of 1861, he was made brigade surgeon and became, according to the author, "the originator of the modern hospital ship." His observations about excessive use of calomel to Surgeon

General Hammond, while both were traveling on the *D. A. January,* led to Hammond's removal of that drug from the army supply table (formulary). He had many other complaints about military medicine, including the lack of skill of Union surgeons and the practice of giving quinine with whiskey. In 1864, he transferred to New York, where he supervised medical evacuation and also the construction of the U.S.S. *J. K. Barnes,* which was, according to the author, the first ship built from the keel up for use as a hospital vessel. During the War, he broke his leg when a fight broke out on a wharf during the loading of wounded soldiers.

Holland, Mary A. Gardner. *Our Army Nurses: Interesting Sketches, Addresses, and Photographs of Nearly One Hundred Women Who Served in Hospitals and on Battlefields during the Civil War.* Boston: B. Wilkins and Co., 1895, 548 p. Reprint. Boston: Lounsberry, Nichols, and Worth, 1897, 600 p.

The book contains brief summaries of ninety-two women who served the Union sick and wounded. Most are written by the individuals themselves and are accompanied by photographs of them in later life. The experiences of these women are individually uninspiring, but their cumulative impact is quite moving.

Holley, Howard L. *The History of Medicine in Alabama.* Birmingham: University of Alabama Press, 1982, 418 p.

This history of Alabama medicine contains a chapter on the Civil War. The book lists all known Confederate military hospitals in Alabama and includes a section on hospitals relocated to Alabama from Georgia after the fall of Atlanta.

Horsman, Reginald. *Josiah Nott of Mobile: Southerner, Physician, and Racial Theorist.* Baton Rouge: Louisiana State University Press, 1987, 348 p.

Josiah Nott was a well-known physician at the time of secession, which he favored. He was recognized as an expert on racial differences; he advanced the theory that the different human races were genetically so different that they could not be descendents from the same individuals. Nott was present at First Manassas as a civilian and helped treat the wounded. "The Minnie balls make such terrible wounds," he said of this experience. He joined the Confederate Medical Department late in 1861 and was made medical director of the army hospital in Mobile, his home. In July of 1862, he inspected the hospital support system for the western armies. The hospitals were located along the Mobile and Ohio Railroad, running from Mobile to Tupelo, Mississippi. They utilized excessive and unused medical resources when the Army of Tennessee shifted its base to Chattanooga. Nott was assigned as a staff officer to General Braxton Bragg during the invasion of Kentucky and performed field surgery at the Battle of Perryville.

During the last two years of the War, Nott was director of the Confederate medical facilities in Mobile. In January of 1864, Mobile held five military hospitals with 600 beds. During the year, four additional military hospitals were open; one of these was for sick and injured black workers assigned to the army. He was present during the battle and surrender of Mobile in April of 1865. His duties as a military medical officer were not quite over. On 25 May, the Union ammunition depot in Mobile exploded, killing 200 people. Many of those injured were black Union soldiers. Nott and other Mobile civilian physicians aided in the treatment of the injured, and Union army doctor J. C. Richards wrote a letter to the local newspaper thanking them. Two sons served in the Confederate army: Henry Nott died of typhoid fever in 1862, and James Nott was killed in action at Chickamauga.

Houck, Peter W. *A Prototype of a Confederate Hospital Center in Lynchburg, Virginia.* Lynchburg, VA: Warwick House Publishing, 1986, 228 p.

This book is a detailed history of the Confederate medical activities in Lynchburg, Virginia, with separate chapters on hospitals, diseases, doctors, women, chaplains, and attendants. The author covers everything that happened medically in Lynchburg from the present status of buildings used as hospitals to the exact locations within the local cemetery where the people mentioned in the book are buried.

Houck, Peter W. "A Healing Place." *Civil War: The Magazine of the Civil War Society* 9 (May–June 1991): 40–43.

This article describes the hospital system in Lynchburg, Virginia. It had become a large hospital center by May of 1864 when it was sorely tested after the Battle of the Wilderness. Rail-lines from the battlefield to Richmond had been cut, and the wounded were evacuated to Lynchburg. The author concludes that the Lynchburg hospital system was a Southern success story.

Hubbs, G. Ward. "John B. Read's Okra Paper." *Alabama Review* 43 (1990): 289–96.

John B. Read graduated in medicine from the University of Louisiana at New Orleans in 1842. He spent the war in Alabama, where he worked on the possibility of making paper from the products of the okra plant. He obtained a United States patent for his process just after the War on 26 December 1865.

Hume, Edgar Erskine. "Chimborazo Hospital, Confederate States Army, America's Largest Military Hospital." *Virginia Medical Monthly* 61 (1934): 189–95.

Early in 1862, General Joseph E. Johnston expected a Federal attack upon his force in Manassas. He notified Surgeon General Moore that he was clearing his field hospitals of sick; 9,000 sick soldiers should be hospitalized in Richmond. Moore had only 2,500 beds available, so he took over the barracks on Chimborazo Hill near Richmond and began construction of additional wooden pavilions. He obtained the wood from the now empty tobacco factories of Grant and of Mayo; wood originally intended for tobacco crates was available because tobacco was no longer being shipped abroad. The tobacco factory workers provided much of the labor for the pavilions.

In the first week, 2,000 patients were received and in the next week 2,000 more. Moore appointed a noted Richmond physician, Dr. James Brown McCaw, medical director of Chimborazo Hospital. He had been born in Richmond in 1823; in 1844, he graduated from the University of the City of New York where he took an apprenticeship with the noted surgeon Valentine Mott. He practiced in Richmond where he edited the *Virginia Medical and Surgical Journal,* which stopped publication in 1861. Just before the War, he became Professor of Chemistry at the Medical College of Virginia.

Chimborazo was officially a separate army post with McCaw the post commandant. He had an officer of the line and thirty guards under his command. The hospital had at any one time about forty-five doctors and about forty-five female matrons. The hospital received no extra funds, only the money that the patients would have required for their rations had they been with their regular commands. The hospital owned its own livestock, up to 200 cows and 500 goats, and grazed them on donated land. The boatman Lawrence Lottier guided the vessel called the *Chimborazo* as far as Lexington and Lynchburg to obtain food for the patients from local farmers. According to Hume, during the War, a total of 76,000 patients were admitted to Chimborazo. Of these about 17,000 were wounded and the remainder were sick. Just over 9 percent of these patients died.

When Richmond was evacuated on 2 April 1865, McCaw stayed behind with the patients. The first Federal unit to arrive was the brigade of General Godfrey Weitzel, whose chief surgeon was

Alexander Mott. Mott immediately recognized the doctor who had been apprenticed to his father in New York two decades earlier. McCaw was immediately offered a commission in the Union army with an appointment to continue as medical director of Chimborazo, now under Union control. He declined the offer, but remained as unofficial medical director. During World War I, the chief surgeon of the American Expeditionary Force in France was Walter Drew McCaw, son of James B.

Hume, Edgar Erskine. "The Foundation of American Meterology by the United States Army Medical Department." *Bulletin of the History of Medicine* 8 (1940):202–38.

The author reviews the major role played by the Medical Department of the Army in the development of meterology, especially in the years just before the Civil War. At each army post, the doctor was responsible for making weather observations three times a day (usually actually performed by the hospital steward). The Surgeon General's Office then collated these reports from all over the continent.

Hume, Edgar Erskine. *Ornithologists of the United States Army Medical Corps.* Baltimore: John Hopkins Press, 1942, 583 p.

This book discusses the careers of United States Army officers, mainly doctors, who collected and interpreted bird specimens. Their contributions to ornithology were largely part of their official duties as scientific officers of various expeditions to the Far West. The list of army ornithologists includes many with subsequent Civil War service, both North and South: Crawford, Finley, Foard, Hammond, Irwin, W. S. King, Peters, Prentiss, Sternberg, and E. P. Vollum.

Hutchinson, John F. "Rethinking the Origins of the Red Cross." *Bulletin of the History of Medicine* 63 (1989): 557–78.

The author wishes to counter the "heroic myth" that the International Red Cross was solely the product of Henry Dunant. The idea that both sides in any war were responsible for the humane treatment of all wounded developed from many sources. It was mainly driven by the change from armies made of mercenaries—the scum of the continent—to armies representative of the citizenry. Both ordinary people and rulers worried about the health of soldiers when they were "us" rather than paid mercenaries. The United States Sanitary Commission and other similar organizations had some influence on the development of the Red Cross, but did not effect the growing idea that all medical personnel should be considered neutral noncombatants, not subject to capture or interference with their medical duties. "The Americans, for all the stupendous achievements of the Sanitary Commission," the author concludes, "had nothing to teach the Europeans about the neutralization of hospitals or medical personnel." The reviewer wonders what Hunter Holmes McGuire would say about that.

I

Ingersoll, L. D. *A History of the War Department of the United States.* Washington, DC: Francis B. Mohun, 1880, 613 p.

This history contains separate evaluations of the ten different sections of the War Department. The emphasis is upon the legal statutes that authorize this or that action. A valuable aspect of this work is the clear presentation of the authorized number of personnel of the Medical Department, exclusive of regimental surgeons and assistant surgeons. In 1861, the Medical Department had a surgeon general, thirty surgeons and eighty-three assistant surgeons. In 1862, the Medical Department was authorized one surgeon general with the rank of brigadier general, forty surgeons with the rank of major, and 104 assistant surgeons (or whom twenty-eight held a rank equivalent to captain and the remainder equivalent to first lieutenant). In addition, the Medical Department was authorized 158 surgeons of volunteers; this was a new rank designed for physicians who could serve directly under the surgeon general without being assigned to a regiment. These doctors, with a rank equivalent to major, served in general hospitals or with field armies in brigade or division hospitals. In 1863, the Medical Department was assigned, in addition, one assistant surgeon general with the rank of colonel, one medical inspector-general with the rank of colonel, sixteen medical inspectors, six medical storekeepers, and an additional number of volunteer surgeons and assistant surgeons.

Irons, Gordon V. "Howard College as a Confederate Military Hospital." *Alabama Review* 9 (1956): 22–32.

In the spring of 1863, Marion Hospital in Marion, Alabama, was unable to handle the load of sick and wounded. The Confederate Medical Bureau rented the two dormitories of Howard College. From its founding in August 1863 to December 1864, the Howard College Hopsital admitted 406 patients. Irons based his study upon the admission book, listing all patients and their treatment, and upon an interview with a blank woman nurse, Willie Banks, who was still living in 1955. Almost all drugs were available except that Howard College Hospital frequently ran out of quinine.

J

Jacobs, Joseph. "Some of the Drug Conditions during the War Between the States, 1861–5." *Southern Historical Society Papers* 33 (1905): 161–87.

The author was a pharmacist in Atlanta and based this paper on his discussions with older pharmacists throughout the South who had been druggists during the War, including Crawford W. Long of Athens, Georgia. One section includes a list of anecdotes: the woman who smuggled drugs under her skirt, quinine in letters delivered from the North by the Adams Express Company, and the field promotion of Dr. Cowan by General Forrest because of the success of a home remedy for diarrhea (Epsom salts, bicarbonate of soda, and laudanum dissolved in water). He says that quinine at one point cost $100 an ounce. He gives a table of substitutions for quinine and other drugs.

James, Janet Wilson. "Writing and Rewriting Nursing History: A Review Essay." *Bulletin of the History of Medicine* 58 (1984): 568–84.

This essay reviews eight recent books on the history of nursing. The writer mentions the American Civil War only when discussing a bibliographic volume.

Johns, Frank S., and Anne Page Johns. "Chimborazo Hospital and J. B. McCaw, Surgeon-in-Chief." *Virginia Magazine of History and Biography* 62 (1954): 190–200.

This brief article surveys how Chimborazo Hospital was built and run. The hospital had its own boat, called the *Chimborazo,* which ran up the James River to obtain supplies from farmers. McCaw had read about the utopian communities of the early nineteenth century and based his hospital organization upon their successes and failures. The article includes a contemporary map of the hospital and the location of its records in the National Archives. One case history is given in detail. After much exhausting treatment, the patient finally died and, after the last note in the record, the surgeon has penned: "war is hell."

Jones, Gordon W. "Wartime Surgery." *Civil War Times Illustrated* 2 (May 1963): 7.

This article is an excellent description of the surgery of wounds. Almost every doctor did minor surgery such as lancing boils, but only a few Civil War doctors performed major operations such as amputations. The author describes wartime operations clearly in lay language. He describes, for example, two types of amputations: the guillotine method, in which a slice across the limb cut skin, muscle, and bone, and the more difficult flap method, in which the bone was cut more proximally than other tissues and the muscles covered the bony stump. He concludes that there was "little difference in techniques and skills between the medical departments of the two armies." The author includes Union army statistics from the *Medical and Surgical History* as well as many specific case reports.

Jones, Gordon W. "The Medical History of the Fredericksburg Campaign: Course and Significance." *Journal of the History of Medicine and Allied Sciences* 18 (1963): 241–56.

The author considers Fredericksburg to have been "a turning point in the care of the wounded," when the Letterman system went into full effect.

Jones, Gordon W. "Sanitation in the Civil War." *Civil War Times Illustrated* 5 (November 1966): 12–18.

This essay argues that the lack of knowledge of germ theory, plus the human (especially the male) tendency toward carelessness, multiplied the misery of the War. The author has analyzed the diseases listed in the *Medical and Surgical History*. Fevers called variously typhoid, continued, or sometimes even typhus, were really typhoid fever. From an analysis of autopsy reports, the author is confident that many soldiers had amebic dysentery, some with liver abcesses. Most of the cases of jaundice he thinks were due to viral hepatitis. He thinks that nonspecific diarrhea would be better classified as enteritis. All of these diseases travel from one victim to another through fecal contamination of food and water.

The author has analyzed army regulations concerning sanitation and concludes that, if followed, they would have prevented these contamination diseases. But "sanitation was accepted reluctantly by soldiers because the reasons for its value were unknown. The benefit was merely an empirically observed fact [especially from the Crimean experience]." Asiatic cholera did not occur during the Civil War, although some physicians incorrectly made this diagnosis. A rampant cholera epidemic "at any time during the war could have ended hostilities in a matter of weeks."

Jones, James B., Jr. "Municipal Vice: The Management of Prostitution in Tennessee's Urban Experience. Part I: The Experience of Nashville and Memphis, 1854–1917." *Tennessee Historical Quarterly* 50 (1991): 33–41.

Various efforts were made to decrease the incidence of venereal disease in Memphis and Nashville. Union military authorities in Nashville first attempted forced removal of all prostitutes. When this failed, legalization of prostitution was undertaken. The military Provost Marshal issued a certificate which read: "License is hereby granted to [name written in], a Public Woman, to pursue her avocation in the City of Nashville, Tenn., she having received a Surgeon's Certificate of soundness." A preliminary version of this article was published in *Civil War History* 31 (1985): 270–76.

Jones, Katharine M. *Heroines of Dixie: Confederate Women Tell Their Story of the War.* Indianapolis, IN: Bobbs-Merrill, 1955, 430 p.

This work is a series of vignettes about Confederate women, including a few nurses. The stories are generally excerpts from published reminiscences, such as those of Phoebe Pember and Kate Cumming, but a few of the selections are taken from manuscript collections. Mrs. Mary H. Johnstone wrote to Confederate Vice-President Alexander H. Stephens on 3 February 1862, complaining about the filthy condition of the camps and regimental hospitals in Manassas. She thinks that the problem is that "surgeon appointments remain a political preferment."

Jordan, Ervin L. *Charlottesville and the University of Virginia in the Civil War.* Lynchburg, VA: H. E. Howard, 1988, 225 p.

A chapter on the Charlottesville General Hospital, directed by University of Virginia professor James L. Cabell, is based upon extensive research in primary sources.

Jordan, Philip D. "The Career of Henry M. Farr, Civil War Surgeon." *Annals of Iowa* 44 (1978): 191–211.

Henry M. Farr was born in Huntington, Vermont, in 1828 and graduated from Castleton Medical College, Castleton, Vermont, in 1855. He moved to Salem, Iowa, and married his cousin. At the start of the War, he sold his farm and joined the 25th Iowa as assistant surgeon. Through most of 1862, he was on detached service, in charge of a section of the Keokuk General Hospital. He rejoined the 25th Iowa in time for the Georgia campaign, the capture of Atlanta, and the march to the sea. He was left in Savannah after Sherman's troops went on into South Carolina. He practiced medicine in Mount Pleasant, Iowa, after the War and died in 1921.

K

Kass, Edward H. "History of the Specialty of Infectious Diseases in the United States." *Annals of Internal Medicine* 106 (1987): 745–56.

Although this article covers the era before the Civil War and discusses the postwar contributions of veterans such as Sternberg, the War itself is never specifically mentioned.

Katz, Joel, and Ronald Melzack. "Pain Memories in Phantom Limbs: Review and Clinical Observations." *Pain* 43 (1990): 319–36.

This article reviews modern knowledge of the neurological basis that explains how a person can feel his fingers or toes after his limb has been amputated. The authors credit Silas Weir Mitchell with the first use of the term "phantom limb."

Kenney, Edward C. "From the Log of the *Red Rover,* 1862–1865." *Missouri Historical Review* 60 (1965): 31–49.

The author, retired from his position as Surgeon General of the United States Navy, reviews the career of the first hospital transport. He quotes extensively from correspondence between Surgeon General William Whelan and the medical officers of the *Red Rover:* George H. Bixby, senior medical officer throughout the War, his assistant, George H. Hopkins, and fleet surgeons Edward Gilchrist and Ninian A. Pinkney. Although fitted out as a hospital steamer, the *Red Rover* was armored and had a single 32 pound gun. She was present during the battle of the Western Flotilla against the *C.S.S. Arkansas.* On 29 August 1862, the *Red Rover* caught fire but this was extinguished with help from the nearby *Benton.*

The *Red Rover* received assistance from shore naval hospitals; the first was organized in the Mound City Hotel and the second in the Commercial Hotel in Memphis (later named the Hospital Pinkney). During the course of the War, the *Red Rover* evacuated 2,497 sick and wounded soldiers and sailors. Mortality information is available for the first two and one half years of service; of the first 1,697 patients transported, only 157 died.

Key, Jack D. "U.S. Army Medical Department and Civil War Medicine." *Military Medicine* 133 (1968): 181–92.

This excellent brief review of Union army medicine emphasizes the Army of the Potomac and its four medical directors: W. S. King to August 1861, Charles Tripler to July 1862, Jonathan Letterman to January 1864, and Thomas McParlin.

Key, Jack D. *William Alexander Hammond, M.D.* Rochester, MN: Davies, 1979, 84 p.

This brief survey of Hammond's life includes a bibliography of his publications.

Kimball, Maria Brace. *A Soldier-Doctor of Our Army: James P. Kimball, Late Colonel and Assistant Surgeon-General, U.S. Army.* Boston: Houghton Mifflin, 1917, 192 p.

This book by his widow emphasizes the postwar career of Dr. James P. Kimball, but does include a chapter on his Civil War experiences. During the summer of 1864, Kimball, still a medical student, was assigned as a medical cadet at McDougall Hospital, Fort Schuyler, New York. His duties included the dressing of minor wounds and keeping the register of patients. He noted that most of the soldiers "don't make as much fuss at having a leg or arm amputated as I have seen in civil life at the drawing of a tooth." Kimball attended Albany Medical College because their graduation was in December 1864, allowing him to immediately become assistant surgeon of the 121st New York and join the regiment in the lines before Petersburg. He took part in the Battle of Hatcher's Run, 5 to 7 February 1865. Kimball wrote his mother: "We merely applied temporary dressings, arresting hemorrhages, etc., saw them put into ambulances and sent to the rear." He worked most of the night until he was quite exhausted, but then, he later told his wife, had to work further on wounded Confederates. Kimball was only twenty-five when he was present at Lee's surrender at Appomattox.

King, Joseph E. "Shoulder Straps for Aesculapius: Atlanta Campaign." *Military Surgeon* 114 (1954): 296–306.

In the early winter of 1864, the medical authorities of Sherman's three armies prepared for a spring campaign. Six months of medical supplies were accumulated; new doctors underwent a special training course in treating gunshot wounds, regimental hospitals were consolidated into brigade hospitals; and the best surgeons, regardless of military rank, were appointed to surgical panels. The campaign is divided into battles and advances, but, to the medical officers, it was one long stream of sick and wounded. After about a month of campaigning, the brigade hospitals were further consolidated into division hospitals, each with a special operating panel of the five best surgeons in the division. Each corps developed its own hospital system, as did each of the three armies. The armies of the Cumberland and the Tennessee had their own hospital trains, but the Army of the Ohio had to ship its wounded north to Chattanooga in boxcars (this made Medical Director Hewitt very mad). Even though Sherman's forces were fairly healthy, two out of three soliders undergoing medical evacuation were sick; only one of three was wounded. The single greatest clinical problem was subclinical scurvy, called the "scorbutic taint." The author makes much use of quotations from the *Official Records*.

King, Joseph E. "Shoulder Straps for Aesculapius: Vicksburg Campaign in 1863." *Military Surgeon* 114 (1954): 216–26.

The author attributes the greater medical success of the Vicksburg campaign, as compared to the Peninsula campaign, to the greater organizational capacity of the military commander. The author divides the campaign, medically, into two parts. In the first part, a huge treatment and evacuation system used a great number of steamers to transfer sick and wounded to northern river ports, especially to Memphis. In the second part, Grant had moved below Vicksburg, and such evacuation was not possible. In this phase, Grant regularly and purposely left his wounded behind to be treated by the Confederates. Many medical officers were unhappy with this policy, leaving the wounded "to the mercies of the enemy." Fortunately, great cooperation between rebel and Federal physicians occurred. One fully functioning Federal hospital remained behind in Jackson, Mississippi, even though the city was reoccupied by rebel forces. The doctors and more seriously wounded soldiers later moved from Jackson to Federal lines under flag of truce. Grant always recognized the inviolability of rebel medical activities. After the battle of Champion's Hill, he not only allowed Confederate field hospitals to continue functioning, but provided them supplies and four Union physicians to work under Confederate direction.

King, Lester S. *Transformations in American Medicine: From Benjamin Rush to William Osler.* Baltimore: Johns Hopkins University Press, 1991, 268 p.

This work analyzes the changes in medical thinking that occurred during the nineteenth century. King uses the example of fevers to show that, throughout the nineteenth century, medical thinking gradually changed its intellectual base. "Fever" as a concept of bodily dysfunction had developed into "the fevers" as different diseases. The first differentiation was based upon clinical observations, such as whether a fever was intermittent or continuous. The intermittent fevers, now known to be different forms of malaria, responded to quinine, which was considered a "specific" therapy because it was not of value in all fevers. The second differentiation was based upon autopsy findings; typhoid fever produced specific lesions within the abdomen, while typhus did not. A third differentation, occurring after the Civil War, was based upon different organisms separated by bacteriologic science. Although this work never examines the Civil War, it illuminates the medical mind of the Civil War doctor.

Klawans, Harold L. "The Court-Martial of William A. Hammond." In his *The Medicine of History from Paracelsus to Freud,* pp. 107–26. New York: Raven Press, 1982.

This essay briefly summarizes Hammond's career before and after his court-martial. After a detailed recitation of the charges, the author concludes that "anyone who reviews the case without prejudice" will find that Hammond was either completely innocent or, at the worst, "a little less than circumspect."

Kramer, Howard D. "The Effect of the Civil War on the Public Health Movement." *Mississippi Valley Historical Review* 35 (1948): 449–62.

The movement for sanitation in the 1850s, led by such people as Lemuel Shattuck, was transformed by the Civil War into a desire to maintain healthy armies. This effort, predominately a Northern one, was successful by two measures: (1) the percentage of the troops sick or died of sickness was much less in the Civil War than in previous long wars such as the Crimean War; and (2) the peacetime United States Army in the late 1860s was considerably healthier than the peacetime army of the 1850s. These successes led to a rejuvenated postwar public health movement. "The Shattuck plan of 1850 had been shattered on the rocks of professional apathy and public indifference; by 1865 the sanitary lessons taught by the war were well known to both the people and the medical profession."

Kuykendall, Rhea. "Surgeons of the Confederacy: Arthur R. Barry." *Confederate Veteran* 34 (1926): 209–10.

After a brief period at Chimborazo Hospital, Barry served in the field with the 9th Virginia. He was brigade surgeon at the time of Pickett's charge at Gettysburg. Barry remembered the last words of his brigade commander, Lewis Armistead, as: "Set up your hospital, you will soon have much to do."

L

La Garde, Louis A. *Gunshot Injuries: How They Are Inflicted, Their Complications and Treatment.* New York: William Wood,

1914, 398 p. Reprint. With an introduction by Martin L. Fackler. Mount Ida, AR: Lancer Militaria, 1991, 457 p.

Written for use in World War I, this treatise on gunshot wounds contains many historical comments, comparing contemporary to mid-nineteenth-century treatments. The characteristics of minie balls are described. A case report, including radiography, is presented of a Union soldier wounded 10 May 1864 who had the ball removed by the author on 26 June 1902. In the introduction to the reprint, Fackler points out that modern rifled weapons, using full metal jacket ammunition, rip through human tissue at a high velocity, destroying only what is in their direct path. They thereby cause *less severe* wounds than the lead bullets, especially the minie balls, of the Civil War that expanded when striking flesh.

Lamb, Daniel S. "History of the Army Medical Museum." *Military Surgeon* 53 (1923): 89–140.

This excellent description of the early days of the Army Medical Museum contains extensive quotations from contemporary orders, circulars, and official correspondence. John H. Brinton was the first official Curator. He and J. J. Woodward gathered statistical material for the *Medical and Surgical History* and physical objects for the Museum. Assistant Surgeon Edward Curtis joined the staff in 1864, in charge of microscopic specimens. The first two artists were A. Pohlers and E. Stauch; they visited hospitals and painted from life, as well as drew from photographs. A most important staff member was Frederick Schafhirt, who, with his son, Adolph, prepared bone specimens. Schafhirt had performed this same task for many years, preparing specimens for the anatomical cabinet (medical museum) of the University of Pennsylvania. As he worked, Schafhirt hummed and sang patriotic and romantic German songs. One of the first visitors to the museum was the chief surgeon of the Russian fleet, visiting the United States during the winter of 1863–64; he was impressed with the specimens, although he spent most of his visit studying indian weapons. The author joined the Museum staff in November, 1865.

Lammers, Pat, and Amy Boyce. "Alias Franklin Thompson: A Female in the Ranks." *Civil War Times Illustrated* 22 (January 1984): 24–30.

Sarah Emma Emmonds, disguised as a male named Franklin "Ned" Thompson, became a private in the 2nd Michigan. She, still in the male disguise, was detached to serve as a nurse in Washington hospitals. She helped succor the wounded on the field at the First Battle of Bull Run, was almost captured, and walked twenty

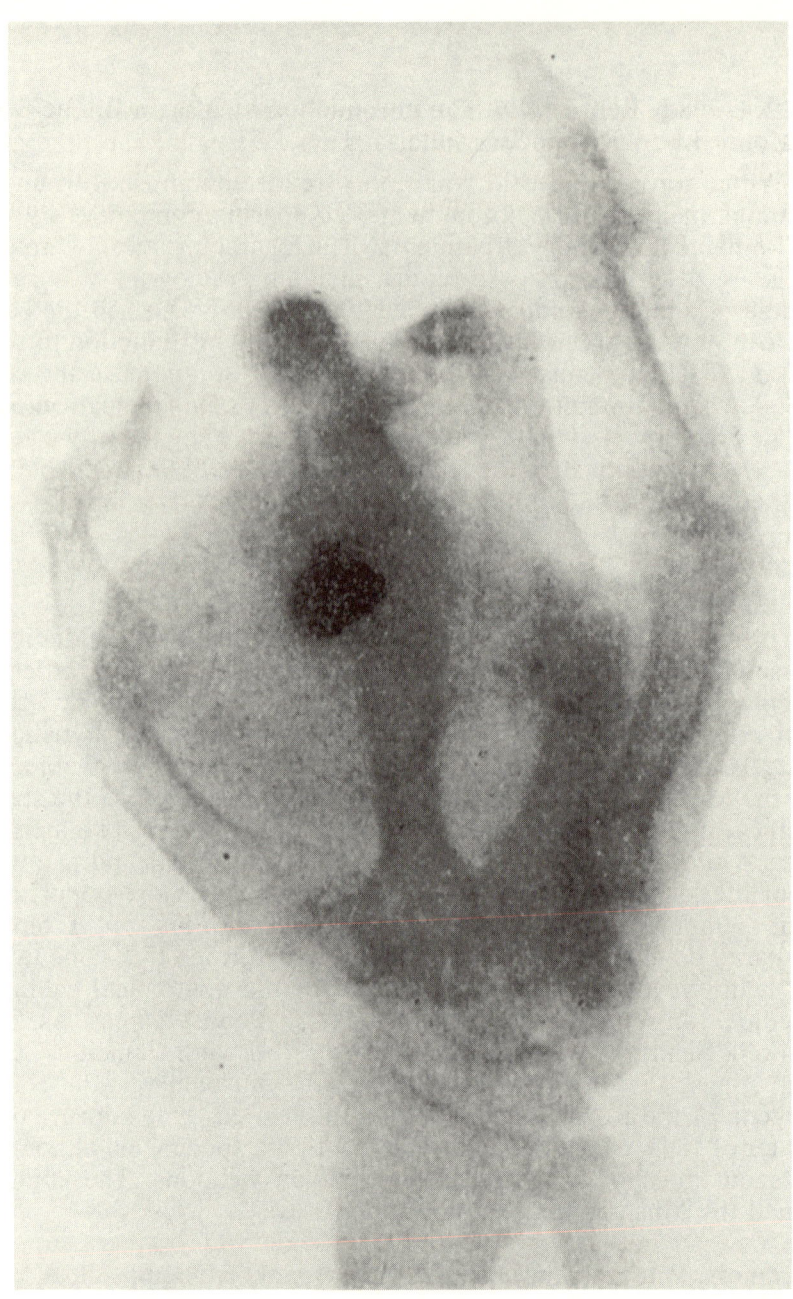

At the Battle of Spottsylvania in May of 1864, a Confederate minie ball struck the upraised hand of Private James M. Denn of the 95th Pennsylvania. Many small bones were shattered and the hand became almost useless for the rest of his life. In 1902, he found a use for his damaged hand while living at the Old Soldier's Home. He would amaze visitors by shaking his hand very vigorously near their ears; they could hear the rattle of a minie ball. Louis A. La Garde, a leading military surgeon, took a radiograph and saw the minie ball still in place after thirty-eight years. Bowing to the ancient surgical principle, "if it is abnormal, cut it out," he removed the ball. This was the last surgical operation of the American Civil War. From La Garde, *Gunshot Injuries*, 1914, p. 387.

miles back to Washington. She became disheartened with nursing after a boyhood friend was killed on the Peninsula; she then entered her second and more exciting career as a spy. The authors of this work seem to believe unflinchingly all the implausible exploits described by Emmonds in her book.

LaPointe, Patricia M. "Military Hospitals in Memphis, 1861–1865." *Tennessee Historical Quarterly* 42 (1983): 325–42.

This very excellent review of Memphis hospitals is based upon a close reading of Memphis newspapers. The Confederates organized 1,200 hospital beds in the city. Later, the Union made Memphis into the major administrative and supply base for the conquest of Vicksburg. Most of the major buildings and many of the churches formed a huge hospital complex of 5,000 beds under the command of Dr. B. J. D. Irwin.

Lattimer, John K. "The Stabbing of Lincoln's Secretary of State on the Night the President Was Shot." *Journal of the American Medical Association* 192 (1965): 107–14.

This article is a detailed medical analysis of the stab wounds suffered by Secretary of State William H. Seward.

Lattimer, John K. *Kennedy and Lincoln: Medical and Ballistic Comparisons of Their Assassinations.* New York: Harcourt Brace Jovanovich, 1980, 378 p.

The first half of this work describes the assassination of President Lincoln in minute detail: type of firearm, path of the wound (unsure), doctors in attendance, and autopsy results. The author concludes that modern medicine could not have saved Lincoln, although immediate tracheal intubation and respiratory support could have produced what the author calls a decerebrate vegetable.

Leech, Margaret. *Reveille in Washington, 1860–1865.* New York: Harper, 1941, 38 p.

This extremely well-written book on life in the Northern capital during the War includes a chapter on hospitals entitled: "The Great Army of the Wounded."

Lester, Richard I. *Confederate Finance and Purchasing in Great Britain.* Charlottesville: University Press of Virginia, 1975, 267 p.

This book describes how the Confederacy obtained materials abroad. Purchasing agents were instructed that medical supplies were second only to arms and powder in importance. Late in the

War, supplies were purchased with cotton; in March of 1864, the Confederate Medical Department had an account of 328 bales available to pay for medicines.

Levin, Beatrice. "Famed Civil War Nurse Mary Bickerdyke Was Better Known to Her Grateful Patients as Mother Bickerdyke." *America's Civil War* 3 (November 1990): 8.

The magazine contains a series on unusual and dynamic "personalities" of the Civil War. Mother Bickerdyke certainly fits both criteria. This brief note describes her major activities and accomplishments.

Levine, Peter. "Draft Evasion in the North during the Civil War." *Journal of American History* 67 (1981): 816–34.

Starting in July of 1863, the North sent out 776,829 draft notices. However, only 46,347 of these men were ever drafted into the Union army. The others escaped in one of several legal ways: hiring a substitute, paying a commutation of $300 (stopped in March of 1864), volunteering or obtaining a commission in the United States Army or Navy, or failing the physical examination. Levine does not discuss these legal methods, but rather analyzes in detail the 161,244 individuals who did not report for their draft examination. These men escaped the draft illegally and were classified as deserters.

Lewis, Samuel E. "Dr. Samuel P. Moore: The Surgeon General of the Confederate States." *Southern Historical Society Papers* 29 (1901): 273–79.

In this brief biographical sketch, reprinted from the *Southern Practitioner,* Dr. Lewis summarizes the life of Surgeon General Moore. He describes Moore as tall, "of soldierly bearing" with features "subdued by thought and studious habits." The author confides that Moore was "greatly distressed in mind" at the time of secession and decided to join the Confederate army only after much anguish. The sketch briefly summarizes Moore's wartime accomplishments. The Association of Army and Navy Surgeons of the Confederate States receives a great deal of attention; all its officers are listed. Moore died at his residence at 202 West Grace Street, Richmond, on 31 May 1889. The sketch lists his descendants.

Lewis, Samuel E. "General T. J. Jackson and his Medical Director, Hunter McGuire, M.D., at Winchester, May, 1862." *Southern Historical Society Papers* 30 (1902): 226–36.

This article briefly describes Hunter Holmes McGuire's action at Winchester in May of 1862. He convinced Jackson to release seven captured Union army doctors on their promise to "use our best efforts" to obtain the release of seven Confederate doctors that might be or become Union prisoners and, furthermore, to work for the principle that all medical officers taken prisoner while performing their duties should be released. The seven Union doctors were named: J. Burd Peale, brigade surgeon; J. J. Jonson, 27th Indiana; Francis Leland, 2nd Massachusetts; Philip Adolphus, United States Army; Lincoln R. Stone, 2nd Massachusetts; Joseph [actually Josiah] F. Day, Jr., 10th Maine; and Evelyn L. Bissel, 5th Connecticut. A letter from McGuire is included in this essay; it includes the information that McGuire's colleague, Daniel B. Conrad, surgeon of the 2nd Virginia, also strongly advocated the release of the Federal doctors.

Linderman, Gerald F. *Embattled Courage: The Experience of Combat in the American Civil War.* New York: Free Press, 1987, 357 p.

This book examines the courage of the average infantryman in the Civil War, arguing that this courage was quite different than the couragelike qualities required to survive modern combat. The book includes the experience of evacuation to the general hospital. "The demands of courage did not disappear with the soldier's withdrawal from battle," claims Linderman. "Those who reached the military hospital found that though it might offer respite to the body, it seldom permitted any relaxation of the will." The presence of women in the hospital increased the need for the severely wounded or dying soldier to demonstrate his courage. "The [female] nurses' working proposition was the supremacy of the individual will as an extension of courage: Suffering was a refining and properly subduing influence to be borne cheerfully and quietly." Proper deathbed behavior required the dying to issue important last words that the nurse would transcribe and send to his relatives. This is an interesting idea, but does not seem to this reviewer too much different than the courage required by a seriously ill patient in the modern hospital. Most people today want to be beside a loved one at the moment of death or, failing that, to know the details of that death including the last words.

Livermore, Thomas Leonard. *Numbers and Losses in the Civil War in America, 1861–65*. Boston: Houghton Mifflin, 1900. Reprint. Dayton, OH: Morningside Press, 1986, 150 p.

This work estimates the losses, both North and South, in each battle of the War. The author has used the best available official figures and attempted reasonable estimates of casualties when such figures were not available. He spells out all his assumptions and calculations. This work is generally considered the definitive conclusion on the dead, wounded, captured, and missing in each of the major battles of the War.

Lynch, John S. "Medical Treatment, or Lack Thereof, Disabled More Soldiers than Bullets or Cannonballs." *America's Civil War* 4 (September 1991): 10.

This very brief overview of Civil War medicine contains a few errors (the Union hospital for nervous diseases was in Philadelphia, not New York), but, in general, serves as an excellent introduction of the medical problems of the conflict. (The reviewer wonders if the flashy title with its confusing grammar [did medical treatment really disable some bullets and cannonballs?] was chosen by the author.)

Mac, Mc

McCarthy, Colman. "Manassas Battlefield is Not Worth Protecting." *The Washington Post,* 24 July 1988, Section C, p. 8.

The author holds that the Manassas battlefield, including the makeshift hospitals still standing, is "no more than another romanticized and dated war zone, a useless place where the stupidity of military violence was unleashed." He recommends a roadside marker and a shopping mall.

McCullough, Champe C. "The Scientific and Administrative Achievement of the Medical Corps of the U.S. Army." *Scientific Monthly* 4 (1917): 410–27.

While this article concerns mainly recent medical advances such as the control of yellow fever and the building of the Panama Canal, a section examines events of the Civil War. The most notable administrative achievement was the creation of the Letterman system. Scientific achievements including the publication of the *Medical and Surgical History* and the Provost-General-Marshal volume on anthropometry. The studies of Mitchell, Keen, and Moorehouse on nerve injuries and of Da Costa on the irritable heart are mentioned. The only specific surgical accomplishment noted by McCullough was the first excision at the ankle joint, performed by John Shaw Billings on 6 January 1862.

McHenry, Lawrence C., Jr. "Surgeon General William Alexander Hammond." *Military Medicine* 128 (1963): 1199–1201.

The preeminent historian of clinical neurology briefly summarizes Hammond's military career, his postwar career as a neurologist, and his efforts at writing fiction.

McIntosh, Suzanne V. "Competitive to the Last, Aged Union and Confederate Veterans to See Who Would Live Longest." *America's Civil War* 4 (September 1991): 8.

This interesting article reviews the final years of the last Civil War veterans. When the last surviving Confederate soldier applied for treatment at a Veterans Administration clinic, he was almost turned away because he was not a veteran of the *United States* armed forces. He was treated for "humanitarian reasons," according to VA administrators, even though he was not officially eligible.

McMurray, Richard M. *Two Great Rebel Armies: An Essay in Confederate Military History.* Chapel Hill: University of North Carolina Press, 1989, 204 p.

This book compares the Army of Northern Virginia to the Army of Tennessee and attempts to determine why one was so much more successful than the other. The Army of Northern Virginia, McMurray concludes, had better line officers at all levels, more graduates of West Point and the Virginia Military Institute, and had the better senior commander, Robert E. Lee. The author does not examine any medical differences between the two armies, such as easier evacuation to Richmond than to the changing medical support center in the West. He makes no attempt to examine any medical statistics to see if the Army of Northern Virginia had a greater percentage of their sick and wounded returned to duty rather than furloughed or discharged.

McPherson, James M. *The Battle Cry of Freedom: The Civil War Era.* New York: Oxford University Press, 1988, 904 p.

The standard single-volume text on the War includes a major section on medical care.

M

Manning, Wade H. "Surgeons of the Confederacy: John Thompson Darby." *Confederate Veteran* 35 (1927): 141–42.

Dr. Darby, a graduate of Jefferson Medical College, was medical director of the Confederate Department of the West. He later served with the Prussian Army in the Austro-Prussian War of 1866.

Marshall, Helen E. *Dorothea Dix: Forgotten Samaritan.* Chapel Hill: University of North Carolina Press, 1937. Reprint. New York: Russell and Russell, 1967, 298 p.

While this book is mainly about her prewar career, one long chapter concerns Dix during the War. After Bull Run, Miss Dix personally arranged for some of the wounded to be housed in private homes in Alexandria. She purchased an ambulance and supplies with her own money. Miss Dix became so incensed at drunken doctors that she overreacted, according to the author, and tried to force all doctors to totally abstain from alcohol for the duration of the War. An order of October 1863 subtly removed her authority by stating that all female nurses must be approved by her, but be assigned by the Surgeon General. She thought that giving this power to the Medical Department "practically abolished the office of superintendant of nurses." On 11 September 1865, she received a curt official notice that her office was closed, and all nurses were discharged. Miss Dix felt that her "Civil War experience was an unhappy one" and wanted to be remembered for her earlier accomplishments.

Massey, Mary Elizabeth. *Ersatz in the Confederacy.* Columbia: University of South Carolina Press, 1952, 233 p.

This book on attempts by the Confederacy to create goods made scarce by the blockade contains an interesting chapter on drugs and medicine.

Maxwell, William Q. *Lincoln's Fifth Wheel: The Political History of the United States Sanitary Commission.* New York: Longmans Green, 1956, 372 p.

This standard history of the United States Sanitary Commission contains a long section concerning how Hammond became surgeon general.

Meleney, Frank L. *Treatise on Surgical Infections.* New York: Oxford University Press, 1948, 713 p.

In the most extensive survey of bacteriological knowledge about hospital gangrene, the author concludes that it was caused by several bacteria acting together. The clinical syndrome is discussed on pages 12 to 17, bacterial synergism as its cause on pages 437 to 469.

Merillat, Louis A., and Delwin M. Campbell. *Veterinary Military History of the United States*, 2 vols. Kansas City, MO: Haver-Glover Laboratories, 1935, 1,172 p.

Prior to the Civil War, each company of cavalry was assigned an enlisted man (or sometimes a civilian) called a farrier, who was assigned to look after the condition of the horses. In 1861, a new rank was established, a veterinary sergeant, paid $17 a month. A few civilians practiced veterinary medicine; most were born and trained in Europe. Dr. John C. Meyer practiced veterinarian medicine in Cincinnati; he had been born in Switzerland and trained at Vienna, graduating in 1846 and coming to the United States after the failed revolutions of 1848. He offered his services to the United States Army at the start of the Civil War, but was told there was no place for him. He visited cavalry camps near Cincinnati and saw that many of the mounts had the serious horse disease glanders. In 1863, the United States Army established the rank of veterinary surgeon, with a pay rate of $75 per month. These volunteers were assigned to the cavalry or to the section of the Quartermaster Department in charge of mount replacement. In 1864, the War Department issued a supply table of medications for use by veterinarians.

Middleton, William S. "Turner's Lane Hospital." *Bulletin of the History of Medicine* 40 (1966): 14–42.

This long article summarizes the nerve injury studies carried on in Philadelphia by Mitchell, Morehouse, and Keen.

Miles, Wyndham D. *A History of the National Library of Medicine, the Nation's Treasury of Medical Knowledge*. Washington, DC: Government Printing Office, 1982, 531 p.

This official history of the National Library of Medicine contains much material on its origin as the library of the Surgeon General's Office.

Miller, E. B. "A Veterinarian's Notes on the Civil War." *Veterinarian Heritage* 8 (1985): 10 25.

The author reviews the history of veterinarians in the Civil War. He states that the first army veterinarian began service on 3 March 1863. Each regiment of cavalry had one veterinarian, who remained officially a civilian, although he wore a uniform with a horseshoe emblem on the sleeve. There were a total of 232 veterinarians in the War, but they had no channel of communication, no superior except the regimental commander, and no way to even communicate with each other.

Miller, Francis Trevelyan, ed. *Prisons and Hospitals.* Vol. 7 of *The Photographic History the Civil War.* New York: Review of Reviews, 1911, 352 p.

This compilation of photographs contains six chapters on medical care written by Civil War veterans, both North and South. The written material contains many observations not available elsewhere. The bugle call that announced sick call, for example, sounded to the soldiers like: "Come and get your quinine, quinine, quinine; come and get your quinine, qui-i-ni-ine."

Miller, Genevieve. "Social Services in a Civil War Hospital in Baltimore." *Bulletin of the History of Medicine* 17 (1945): 439–59.

This article concerns the activities of the Christian Commission and the Ladies Union Aid Society at the Jarvis United States General Hospital in Baltimore. These groups provided special meals, plays, excursions, and other forms of recreation for convalescents. The overall leader was Mrs. Sarah S. Spear, of Lyme, New Hampshire. Contemporary printed material is appended, including orders for sentries (quite detailed), contracts for cooks (all cooks were black and received $10 per month), a call for donation of old rags "suitable for dressing wounds," and sample menus for Thanksgiving and New Year's dinners.

Moore, Frank. *Women of the War: Their Heroism and Self-Sacrifice.* Hartford, CT: S. S. Scranton, 1867, 596 p.

These descriptions of the efforts of Union women for the Northern cause include nurses and matrons such as Mother Bickerdyke.

Mostofi, F. K. "Contributions of the Military to Tropical Medicine." *New York Academy of Medicine Bulletin* 44 (1968): 702–20.

The author states that the appointment, in June of 1861, by Secretary of War Cameron, of a Commission to Study and Advise on Sanitation in the Army "was one of the most important historical events in our military medical annals." He reviews the accomplishments of Hammond and of the United States Sanitary Commission. Most of the contributions of the United States military to tropical medicine occurred in the post–Civil War period.

Murdock, Eugene C. "Pity the Poor Surgeon." *Civil War History* 16 (1970): 18–36.

This article emphasizes the medical examination to determine if the draftee or volunteer should become a soldier or if the sick and wounded soldier is able to return to full duty. The biggest problem of the fitness for duty examination was dissimulation. The malingerer became expert in the ability to feign specific signs and symptoms.

Murdock, Eugene C. *One Million Men.* Westport, CT: Greenwood Press, 1980, 366 p.

The examination of recruits in the North was performed by physicians hired and supervised by the Provost-Marshall-General Bureau. This book contains immense detail about the result of these examinations.

N

Nevins, Allan. *The War for the Union.* Vol. 1, *The Improvised War;* Vol. 2, *War Becomes Revolution;* Vol. 3, *The Organized War;* and Vol. 4, *The Organized War to Victory.* New York: Scribner's 1959–71, 435, 667, 532, and 448 pages.

This is the best narrative history of the Civil War, written from the Northern point of view. As the volume titles suggest, Nevin thinks that the War recreated the country, changing it from a sprawling confederation of states to an organized modern nation. Medical problems, especially the horror of removing the wounded after battles, are mentioned throughout, but Union medical activities receive special attention in volume 3. The Medical Department can be considered a test case of his thesis, moving from improvisation to organization as the war progressed.

Newsome, Robert I., Jr. "A Kentucky Yankee's Story of Fort Donelson." *Lincoln Herald* 87 (Fall 1985): 73–75.

David Russell was hospital steward of the 17th Kentucky (Union). The author analogizes the Civil War hospital steward to a modern medical corpsman. The article includes a letter from Russell to his father. He describes his activities at the Battle of Fort Donelson. With the surgeon of the 17th Kentucky, Dr. Burgess, Russell set up a regimental hospital or aide station just seventy-five yards behind the battle line. The wounded were brought to the regimental hospital by ten men especially detailed for this duty: Newsome derisively refers to them as "Company Q." Newsome died of diarrhea just two months later.

Noe, Adrianne, and George S. M. Cowan. "Microscopy and the

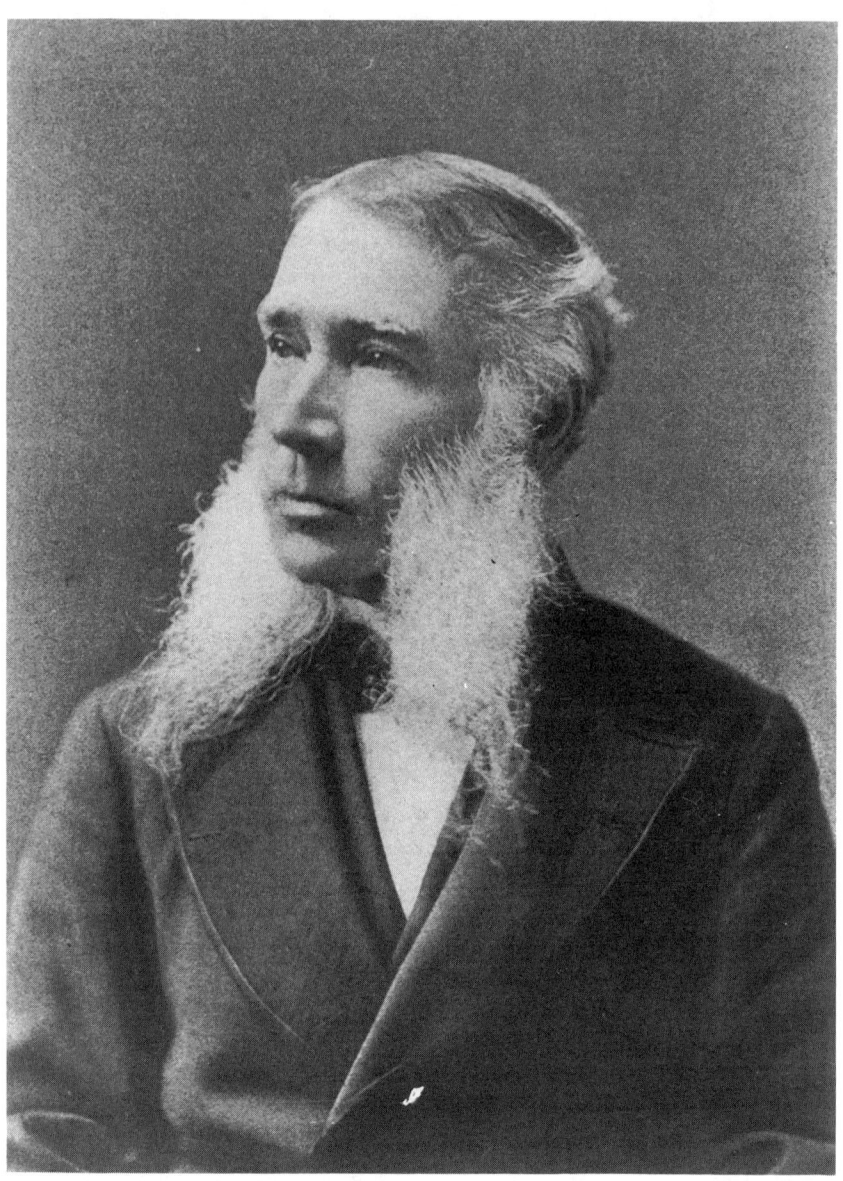

Samuel P. Moore was the surgeon general of the Confederate States Army. He always wore civilian clothes, as in this photograph from Miller's *Photographic History of the Civil War,* and some secondary works claim, incorrectly, that he was a civilian. A famous London tailor made a beautiful Confederate gray uniform for him, but it was captured by the United States Navy. The medical officers under his command thought that he was the perfect leader for the Medical Department of the Confederate States Army. Samuel H. Stout said that Moore was the finest officer he ever met, although he immediately added that he had never met Robert E. Lee. Some thought that his only failing was a tendency to favor form over results. He never raised the ruckus that Hammond did in the Union Medical Department; he served to the end of the War and described in the *Confederate States Medical and Surgical Journal* the dismissal by court-martial of his Union counterpart. Moore tried to obtain cooperation from other Confederate Departments, but was unable to put in place a system analogous to the Letterman system of the North.

Army Medical Museum." *Caduceus: A Museum Quarterly for the Health Sciences* 2 (Summer 1986): 1–37.

This article concerns the Army Medical Museum with emphasis on microscopes and microscopy. The Armed Forces Medical Museum of the Armed Forces Institute of Pathology, Washington, a descendant of the original museum founded by Hammond and nurtured by Brinton, Otis, and Woodward, contains 900 microscopes.

Nolan, David L., and David A. Pattillo. "The Army Medical Department and the Civil War: Historical Lessons for Current Medical Support." *Military Medicine* 154 (1989): 265–71.

This essay contains a brilliant structural analysis of the medical evacuation scheme before and after the development of the Letterman system. The major problem in 1861 was a clash in control between evacuation (Quartermaster Department) and treatment (Medical Department). The major improvement was to move control of ambulances, including training and command of crews, to the Medical Department. The authors fear that recent changes in United States military doctrine are producing a medical evacuation and control system analogous to the 1861 situation.

Norris, John. "The Scurvy Disposition: Heavy Exertion as an Exacerbating Influence on Scurvy in Modern Times." *Bulletin of the History of Medicine* 57 (1983): 325–38.

The author reviews clinical studies that seem to indicate that physical exertion speeds depletion of body stores of vitamin C. He then analyzes the reports of arctic expeditions to show that heavy exertion exacerbates clinical scurvy. He does not mention the Civil War, but his information helps explain why scurvy was so common in some difficult campaigns.

P

Parrish, William E. "The Western Sanitary Commission." *Civil War History* 36 (1990): 17–35.

This article reviews the activities of the Western Sanitary Commission. According to the author, this Commission first suggested the use of hospital boats on the Western rivers. The army obtained the vessels, the Commission outfitted them as hospital ships. The Western Sanitary Commission developed a fairly good working relationship with the United States Sanitary Commission until they began competing for donations in the east. The Western Sanitary

Commission received a good deal of financial support from New England.

Peabody, Charles Newton. *ZAB: (Brevet Major Zabdiel Boylston Adams, 1829–1902, Physician of Boston and Framingham).* Charlottesville: University Press of Virginia, 1984, 255 p.

This book on the life of Zabdiel Adams includes four chapters on his Civil War experiences. He began as assistant surgeon of the 7th Massachusetts and came under fire when removing the wounded during the Peninsula campaign. He was promoted to surgeon of the 32nd Massachusetts and operated for two days and nights during and after the Battle of Gettysburg. He resigned his commission because of failing eyesight. Upon return to Boston and with extended rest, his eye inflammation improved, and he rejoined the army. His second army experience was, however, as a line officer, not as a physician. He was promoted to brevet major of the 56th Massachusetts. He was wounded in the leg at the Battle of the Wilderness and taken prisoner. After exchange, he participated in the siege of Petersburg. This biography quotes extensively from his letters and wartime notes. The author states that Adams is the only physician to be honored with a plaque at the Gettysburg Battlefield Park.

Phalen, James M. "The Life of Charles Stuart Tripler." *Military Surgeon* 82 (1938): 459–63.

Tripler was born in the Bowery, New York. He was apprenticed to a doctor and apothecary, Stephen Brown, and graduated from the College of Physicians and Surgeons in 1827. After a year of residency at Bellevue Hospital, he joined the army. Stationed at West Point, he took some classes with United States Military Academy cadets. This article briefly surveys his army career. Tripler developed a malignant tumor of his neck and died in 1866. The new (1938) general hospital in Honolulu is named for him.

Phalen, James M. "Surgeon Thomas A. McParlin: Letterman's Successor with the Army of the Potomac." *Military Surgeon* 87 (1940): 68–71.

McParlin was born in Annapolis, Maryland, in 1825. He graduated from St. John's College in that city in 1843 and then obtained his medical training at the University of Maryland. He was the medical director for Pope's unsuccessful Army of Virginia; the medical disasters of Second Bull Run were not blamed on him. He was on hospital duty at the Naval School Hospital in Annapolis when he was called to succeed Letterman as medical director of the Army of the Potomac in January 1864. He remained in the army after the War, retiring in 1889. He died in Annapolis in 1897.

Phalen, James M. "Chiefs of the Medical Department, United States Army: Thomas Lawson, Clement Alexander Finley, William Alexander Hammond, Joseph K. Barnes." *Army Medical Bulletin* 52 (1940): 30–51.

As part of a survey of all United States Army Surgeon Generals, Phalen gives brief biographies of the four who served during the Civil War.

Phisterer, Frederick. *Statistical Record of the Armies of the United States*. New York: Charles Scribner's Sons, 1883, 343 p.

This work contains many different military records, statistical and otherwise, but the major interest is the author's thoughtful attempt to calculate total Union army losses in the Civil War. He thinks that the report of the adjutant general is more likely to be correct for the number of soldiers killed in action, while the surgeon general's report is more accurate for those dying of wounds and of disease. The author thinks that these figures are as close to the actual numbers as we can approach:

Killed in action:	44,238
Died of wounds:	49,205
Died of disease:	186,216
Died, unknown cause:	24,184
Other (homicide, suicide, execution):	526
Total deaths, Union army	304,369

The book also presents statistical data on medical discharges and on deaths that occurred in general hospitals.

Pilcher, James E. "Brevet Brigadier General Clement Alexander Finley, Surgeon General of the United States Army, 1861–1862." *Military Surgeon* 15 (1904): 59–66.

The author describes Finley's army career. A major disagreement with Secretary of War Stanton is outlined, based upon the personal recollections of Joseph R. Smith. Finley was a medical graduate of the University of Pennsylvania.

Pilcher, James E. "Brigadier General William Alexander Hammond, Surgeon General of the United States Army, 1862–1864." *Military Surgeon* 15 (1904): 145–55.

This article presents a survey of Hammond's army career, his accomplishments as surgeon general, and his court-martial.

Pilcher, James E. "Brevet Major General Joseph K. Barnes, Surgeon General of the United States Army, 1864–1882." *Military Surgeon* 15 (1904): 219–24.

This article survey Barnes's army career. Barnes was forced to retire by a new law limiting the ages of senior officials and died shortly thereafter. He was a graduate of the University of Pennsylvania and treated both presidents Lincoln and Garfield after they were shot.

Pilcher, James E. "Dr. Samuel Preston Moore, Surgeon General of the Confederate Army, 1861–1865." *Military Surgeon* 16 (1905): 210–15.

This is a laudatory review of Moore's life, with emphasis upon his twenty-five years of service with the old United States Army prior to the Civil War.

Preston, R. A. "A Letter from a British Military Observer of the American Civil War." *Military Affairs* 16 (1952): 49–60.

Edward O. Hewett was a British military officer stationed in Canada. He visited the Army of the Potomac and western Union armies late in 1862. He was accompanied by a British army surgeon, a Dr. Jameson, and made many medical observations. He noted that Union army doctors, unlike contemporary British practice, performed surgery on the wounded where it could be seen by many people, including those about to be operated upon. After Antietam, the British officer saw 3,000 Federal wounded, described as "wretched creatures," laying under trees in a space about 300 yards square. The sixty surgeons, many of whom were French, German, and Irish, were "cutting and sawing more like the devils and machines than human beings." He saw medical cadets fight over discarded limbs to be used for dissection to study anatomy.

Q

Quebbeman, Frances E. *Medicine in Territorial Arizona*. Phoenix: Arizona Historical Foundation, 1966, 424 p.

This review of medical activities in early Arizona is a catalog of doctors, including those military and civilian, North and South, who were in the Territory during the Civil War period.

R

Ramage, James A. "The Wounded of Shiloh." *Civil War: The Magazine of the Civil War Society* 9 (May–June 1991): 10–15.

This article is a very excellent description of the confused medical care at the Battle of Shiloh, with emphasis on the Union experience. Robert W. Murray, a regular army physician, was medical director of Buell's Army of the Ohio. When he arrived on the scene, he took control from Henry S. Hewit, a volunteer physician who was Grant's medical director. They set up tents to house the many wounded and began evacuating them to the north on steamers belonging to a makeshift series of authorities.

Reasoner, M. A. "The Development of the Medical Supply Service." *Military Surgeon* 63 (1928): 4–5.

This brief review discusses how medications, bandages, and other material are supplied; the Civil War is mentioned.

Reverby, Susan M. *Ordered to Care: The Dilemma of American Nursing, 1850–1945*. New York: Cambridge University Press, 1987, 286 p.

This review of American nursing includes four pages on the role of Northern women during the Civil War (male nurses are not mentioned). The author states that hospital matrons "perceived the authority of the physicians and surgeons as their biggest problem." According to the author, the women developed a mode of behavior based on upper-class professionalism and the authority of a mother figure.

Riley, Harris D., Jr. "Medicine in the Confederacy." *Military Medicine* 118 (1956): 53–64 and 144–53.

This excellent brief review quotes frequently from primary sources.

Riley, Harris D., Jr. "General Robert E. Lee: His Medical Profile." *Virginia Medical Monthly* 105 (1978): 495–501.

Lee was robustly healthy until the War. He was seized with chest pain at Chancellorsville in 1863, diagnosed by contemporaries as pericarditis. The author feels that Lee suffered from "generalized vascular disease due to atherosclerosis" from 1863 until his death in 1870 at age sixty-three. During the War, Lee experienced paroxysmal pain in the chest, arm, and back due to angina pectoris, "myocardial insufficiency due to coronary atherosclerosis."

Riley, Harris D., Jr. "Joseph Jones, M.D.: An Early Clinical Investigator." *Southern Medical Journal* 80 (1987): 623–29.

A brief, informative review of the life of Jones, with emphasis on his postwar career.

Riley, Harris D., Jr. "Jefferson Davis and His Health: Part II, January, 1861 to December, 1889." *Journal of Mississippi History* 49 (1987): 261–87.

Davis experienced severe facial pain throughout much of his life, especially when he was under great emotional stress. The author considers a differential diagnosis of this problem; he rejects the diagnosis made by several biographers of tic douloureux (also called trigeminal neuralgia). He believes the most likely diagnosis is facial neuralgia secondary to keratitis with corneal ulceration. Undoubtedly, Davis suffered emotional strain in the years 1864 to 1866 with such symptoms as lack of appetite, insomnia, and weight loss.

Riley, Harris D. Jr. "Medical Furloughs in the Confederate States Army." *Journal of Confederate History* 2 (1989): 115–131.

This article reviews the changing rules that determined how a sick or wounded Confederate soldier could obtain a medical furlough to convalesce at home. Medical furlough was a severe drain upon military manpower. Many of the soldiers sent home for medical reasons could have remained with their commands. An example is John Thomas Graves, a Missouri soldier discharged in 1863 because of poor health. He lived until age 108, dying in 1950.

Riley, Harris D., Jr. "General Richard Taylor, C.S.A.: Louisianian, Distinguished Military Commander, and Author, with Speculations on his Health." *Southern Studies* 1 (1990): 67–86.

This article reviews the major accomplishments of Richard Taylor, son of Zachary, and then examines his medical symptoms. The author argues that Taylor had an attack of rheumatic fever at age twenty and that rheumatic heart disease caused his premature death at age fifty-three. More difficult to explain are Taylor's wartime symptoms of nervous headaches and weakness of both legs. Rheumatic joint pain might be an explanation, or Taylor might have suffered a conversion reaction from the psychological stress of leading men into battle.

Riley, Harris D., Jr., and Amos Christie. "Deaths and Disabilities in the Provisional Army of Tennessee." *Tennessee Historical Quarterly* 43 (1984): 132–54.

A study of the illnesses in the Provisional Army of Tennessee, the nucleus of the force that became the Army of Tennessee, based on the regimental returns in the Tennessee State Archives for the period when the force was under state control.

Rittenhouse, Henry N. "U.S. Army Medical Storekeepers." *American Journal of Pharmacy* 37 (1865): 87–90.

The author describes the role of pharmacists for the Union army during the Civil War. A board of medical officers passed on the qualifications of each person applying for the position of medical storekeeper; only pharmacists had enough knowledge to qualify. They were paid $124.16 per month. They remained civilians and were called "Mr." in civilian establishments and "Captain" if assigned to military units. The author states that pharmacists in this position used their business or accounting knowledge more than their scientific knowledge. A typical action occurred in this manner: a medical officer made a requisition for something he needed, the medical director of his department approved the request, and then the medical storekeeper packed it and sent it to the quartermaster for shipment to the initiating doctor.

Robertson, James I., Jr. *General A. P. Hill: The Story of a Confederate Warrior.* New York: Random House, 1987, 382 p.

This is an excellent military history of the Civil War career of General Ambrose Powell Hill of the Army of Northern Virginia. Hill was sick during the Battle of Gettysburg and, according to some military historians, may not have attacked on the first day with sufficient vigor. He became so ill during the Battle of the Wilderness that he relinquished command of his corps to Jubal Early. He was taken to the battlefield in an ambulance. Robertson attributes his illness, especially his inability to ride a horse, to gonorrheal prostatitis. This interpretation is not in the preface, summary, or index, but is buried in the narrative; gonorrhea on page 12, prostatitis on page 22, and serious sickness at the Wilderness on pages 262 through 268.

Robertson, James I., Jr. *Soldiers Blue and Gray.* Columbia: University of South Carolina Press, 1988, 278 p.

This volume describes the War from the point of view of the ordinary soldier, North and South. One chapter covers sickness, surgery, evacuation, and hospitalization.

Roddis, Louis H. *A Short History of Nautical Medicine.* New York: Paul B. Hoeber, 1941, 359 p.

A doctor in the United States Navy provides a very brief history of medical problems at sea from the ancient world to the present. He emphasizes the American experience and has a major section on the Civil War from the Northern viewpoint. Much of the commentary is a series of stories of individual accomplishments. Assistant Surgeon J. H. Gotwald was serving aboard the U.S.S. *Keystone State* on blockade when Confederate ironclads sortied from Charleston. He was struck and killed by a shell while treating wounded sailors. Naval surgeon William Longshaw, Jr., received accolades for guiding a rowboat from the U.S.S. *Lehigh* to carry a howser to the ironclad U.S.S. *Nahant,* caught on a sandbar. He was under such heavy fire that the howser was cut by a shell, and he had to make a second trip with another. The *Nahant* was pulled free before it could be attacked from the shore. Longshaw was killed in action during the attack on Fort Fisher in January 1865. Before the commissioning of the *Red Rover,* a small shore naval hospital was established at Mound City, Illinois. Later, naval medical authorities established the Pinkney Hospital in Memphis, named for Ninian Pinkney, the dynamic chief naval surgeon on the Western rivers. During the Civil War, a total of thirty-three naval surgeons lost their lives.

Rogers, Margaret Greene. *Civil War Corinth, 1861–1865.* Corinth, MS: privately printed, 1987, 46 p.

This pamphlet describes the city of Corinth during the Civil War, with special reference to modern structures. The Driver House, for example, was used as a hospital by both North and South; it is today the home of O. R. Smith, Jr. During the siege of Corinth by Halleck, the huge Confederate garrison suffered severely from disease. The many soldiers who died were buried in trenches along the Droke Road; the exact location was lost, but the author believes that the present Chamber of Commerce Building is located over the graves.

Rolleston, Humphrey. "History of Cinchona and Its Therapeutics." *Annals of Medical History* 3 (1931): 261–70.

The therapeutic effects of cinchona were probably known to the Incas. By the middle of the seventeenth century, Spaniards were grinding the bark and selling it to treat ague. In the early nineteenth century, attempts were made to transplant the cinchona tree to India, Ceylon, and Java. Although these attempts were later successful, at the time of the American Civil War, all quinine originated in South America.

Roos, Charles A. "Physicians to the Presidents, and Their Patients:

A Biobibliography." *Bulletin of the Medical Library Association* 49 (1961): 291–360.

As part of a series on doctors to presidents, Roos covers the health, shooting, and autopsy of Abraham Lincoln. The publications of the various doctors who were with Lincoln during his last hours are annotated; inconsistencies are recorded. Some of the military doctors who treated Lincoln also treated Garfield after he had been shot.

Rosenberg, Charles E. "Florence Nightingale on Contagion: The Hospital as Moral Universe." In his *Healing and History,* pp. 116–36. New York: Dawson, 1979.

Nightingale mirrored the medical thought of the middle nineteenth century when she considered the human body as a dynamic system interacting with its environment. "Consider," she said, "that an adult exhales by the lungs and skin in 24 hours three pints at least of moisture, loaded with organic matter ready to enter into putrefaction; that in sickness the quantity is often increased, the quality is always more noxious." She recommended most forcefully that the sick should have adequate ventilation and daily bedding changes. Rosenberg points out that this type of ecological thinking was not responsive to the discoveries of bacteriology (one organism, one disease) that occurred in the last decades of the century.

Rosenberg, Charles E. *The Rise of America's Hospital System.* New York: Basic Books, 1987, 437 p.

This is the standard work on the organization of American hospitals to about 1920. At the beginning of the nineteenth century, most medical and surgical therapy occurred in the home. The convalescent was nursed by his female relatives. If surgery was needed, it was performed on the kitchen table. The hospitals that existed were those mainly for people who had no female relatives who could stay home and provide nursing care, marine hospitals for seamen and boatmen too sick to travel with their vessels, post hospitals for soldiers away from home, and city hospitals—often part of the city alms house—that provided convalescent care for transients and the poor. By the end of the century, the more complex surgical procedures were performed in operating suites in the new hospital; female nurses or nursing trainees provided professional nursing care. The Civil War is mentioned, particularly in relation to the development of pavilion hospitals with ventilation, but is not emphasized.

Roster of All the Regimental Surgeons and Assistant Surgeons in the Late War and Hospital Service. Washington, DC: G. M. Van Buren, 1883. Reprint, with an introduction by F. Terry Hambrecht. Gaithersburg, MD: Olde Soldier Books, 1989, 316 p.

This work lists the surgeons, assistant surgeons, and hospital stewards in each volunteer regiment of the Union army. The location of those physicians still alive about 1880 is also given; many have moved west. Not included are brigade surgeons of the volunteer army such as John Brinton and most doctors from the regular army such as Sternberg or Hammond.

Rothstein, William G. *American Medical Schools and the Practice of Medicine: A History.* New York: Oxford University Press, 1987, 408 p.

The author examines medical education, with special reference to its role in medical practice, throughout the history of the United States. He uses these years as organizational breaks: 1825, 1860, 1900, and 1950. In the period after 1860 new developments discussed include clinical medical science, especially bacteriology, the development of surgery, the increasing specialization of medicine, and the growth of higher education in general. The only mention of the American Civil War is the observation that fewer wound infections occurred in hospital tents than in traditional buildings, leading to an emphasis on ventilation in new hospital construction.

Rozear, Marvin P., E. Wayne Massey, Jennifer Horner, Erin Foley, and Joseph C. Greenfield. "Robert E. Lee's Stroke." *Virginia Magazine of History and Biography* 98 (1990): 291–308.

When Robert E. Lee developed a stroke and died after the War, his doctors, R. L. Madison and Howard T. Barton, published a full account of his illness. The present authors review that account in the light of modern medical knowledge. The major conclusion was that Lee could not speak because of the condition of "abulia" or organic listlessness. The authors think that the last words attributed to Lee were concocted by a family friend, William Preston Johnston (son of Albert Sydney).

Rudolph, Ross. "Wound Treatments, Nostrums, and Hokums." In *Chronic Problem Wounds,* edited by Ross Rudolph and Joel M. Noe, pp. 47–51. Boston: Little Brown and Company, 1983.

This essay provides a huge list of materials that have been rubbed into wounds with the aim of healing; most were ineffective, but some are now known to kill bacteria.

Rutkow, Ira M. *The History of Surgery in the United States, 1775–*

1900. Volume I: *Textbooks, Monographs, and Treatises*. San Francisco: Norman Publishing, 1988, 488 p.

This work is an annotated bibliography of surgical works published in the United States. Many texts and handbooks of the Civil War period are included. Rutkow's annotations include detailed information not readily available elsewhere.

Ryons, Fred B. "The United States Army Medical Department, 1861–1865." *Military Surgeon* 79 (1936): 341–56.

At First Bull Run, only one field hospital was established, at Sudley Church. The general hospitals in Centreville had no water: the thirsty troops passing through the town had exhausted the wells, and what little water had been obtained for the hospital was drunk by retreating troops. At Second Bull Run, the medical director, McParlin, had obtained Letterman's plan in writing but had had no time to put it into effect. The author then describes the changes that occurred at Cedar Mountain and Antietam with emphasis on the development of the Letterman system. The author thinks that the ambulance and field hospital system in the Army of the Potomac in 1864 were *better* than the medical organization he saw in the United States Army in the conflicts of 1898 and 1918. "The system of caring for the wounded, devised by Letterman and carried out by McParlin and others, was the basis of all the systems now in use in the great armies of the world."

S

Sabine, David B. "Captain Sally Tompkins." *Civil War Times Illustrated* 4 (November 1965): 36–39.

This brief article summarizes how Sally Tompkins organized and directed the Robertson Hospital in Richmond.

Savitt, Todd L. *Medicine and Slavery: The Diseases and Health Care of Blacks in Antebellum Virginia*. Urbana: University of Illinois Press, 1978, 332 p.

This major survey of the health of blacks just before the Civil War does not cover the medical problems of the black soldiers of the Union Army.

Scaife, William R. *Confederate Surgeon*. Atlanta, GA: privately printed, 1985, 134 p.

Based on printed sources, this book surveys the career of William L. Scaife, assistant surgeon of the 9th Texas. This Confederate doctor, grandfather of the author, was present at Second Manassas, Antietam, Fredericksburg, the Atlanta campaign, and at the Battle of Nashville.

Schildt, John W. *Antietam Hospitals.* Chewsville, MD: Antietam Publications, 1987, 64 p.

This pamphlet describes the buildings—many still standing—used as hospitals by the North and the South during and following the Battle of Antietam.

Schildt, John W. *Hunter Holmes McGuire: Doctor in Gray.* Chewsville, MD: privately printed, 1986, 135 p.

This biography of Stonewall Jackson's medical director includes his postwar career as a major figure in American medicine.

Schullian, Dorothy M., and Frank B. Rogers "The National Library of Medicine." *Library Quarterly* 28 (1958): 1–17 and 95–121.

This review of the development of the Library of the Surgeon General's Office into the National Library of Medicine includes some information about the Civil War. When first catalogued in 1840, the library contained 200 volumes. The first printed catalog, issued on 10 May 1864, listed 1,365 volumes. By the end of the War (the second catalog was dated 23 October 1865), the collection had grown to 2,253 volumes.

Schwartz, L. Laszlo. "The Development of the Treatment of Jaw Fractures." *Journal of Oral Surgery* 2 (1944): 193–221.

The author, an oral surgeon, reviews the history of jaw fractures from the earliest times. The modern treatment of the condition was devised by James Baxter Bean during the American Civil War. Bean was born in Tennessee in 1824 and obtained a medical degree (school unknown). He was practicing medicine and dentistry in Micanopy, Florida, in 1861. In 1864, he visited the Confederate hospitals in Atlanta, offering to treat jaw fractures by his own method without charge. He was so successful that medical inspector E. N. Covey arranged a special dental ward at the military hospital at Macon. About forty patients were treated with Bean's splint, which brought together the split ends of either the upper or lower jaw, holding them together with a complex series of straps until a healing union could occur. The splint was applied only after Bean had taken an impression of the bite and adjusted his apparatus accordingly. In the last months of the War, a special dental ward was located in the Receiving and Way Hospital of Richmond; Bean was not present, but hospital steward W. S. Wilkinson was assigned dental duties, apparently as he had been trained by Bean. James Bolton thought that Bean's splint was excellent if time and resources permitted; for field work he preferred a simpler splint, without the need for a dental impression.

Schwartz, L. Laszlo. "James Bolton (1812–1869): Early Proponent of External Skeletal Fixation." *American Journal of Surgery* 66 (1944): 409–413.

James Bolton was born in Savannah in 1812 and graduated from the College of Physicians and Surgeons, New York, in 1836. In 1864, he was chief surgeon of the Confederate 3rd Corps Receiving Hospital. Following the battles of the Wilderness and of Spotsylvania, he wrote on 29 May 1864 to William A. Carrington, medical director of the hospitals of Richmond. Although Carrington was not his superior, nor even in his chain of command, he begged him to send food and medicine. "I have scant rations for two days. This whole country has been drained of provisions. . . . I have but few articles of medicine and these I am compelled to use sparingly." He attributes the high rate of mortality to these supply problems. (Schwartz found this letter in the National Archives).

Although the author discusses Bolton's difficulties as a senior medical officer, the main thrust of the essay is to evaluate Bolton's article in the *Confederate States Medical and Surgical Journal* entitled "New Method of Treating Ununited Fractures of the Long Bones." Most patients with fractured legs undergo amputation. Bolton thinks legs can be saved in the following manner: the patient is anesthetized, the leg is straightened by "powerful extension," two rods are placed in leg bones on either side of the fracture, and another rod is tightly fastened to these, parallel to the shaft of the fractured bone. This technique prevents the leg from bending and eventually the fracture will heal, saving the leg.

Schwartzman, Robert J., and Toni L. McLellan. "Reflex Sympathetic Dystrophy: A Review." *Archives of Neurology* 44 (1987): 555–61.

This brief article reviews the historical background and modern knowledge concerning the symptomatology encountered by Silas Weir Mitchell in Civil War soldiers.

Senn, Nicholas. "Esculapius on the Field of Battle." In his *Medico-*

Surgical Aspects of the Spanish American War, pp. 340–49. Chicago: American Medical Association Press, 1900.

Senn compares wound surgery as practiced during the American Civil War with the more modern surgery of the Spanish American War. "Aseptic surgery has driven out of our military hospitals the four greatest enemies of the wounded soldier: hospital gangrene, secondary hemorrhage, pyemia, and erysipelas. The probe, an instrument of torture, danger and fallacy, has been abandoned for the X-ray in locating bullets lodged in the body."

Seth, Joseph B. "Surgeons of the Confederacy: Edward N. Covey of Maryland." *Confederate Veteran* 34 (1926): 210.

Edward N. Covey had been an assistant surgeon with the United States Army since 1855. He resigned to serve with the Confederate Army in Arizona and New Mexico. He was captured in the far west in 1862. After exchange, he was in charge of the hospitals in Raleigh, North Carolina; he made an official inspection of the Andersonville prison.

Shaffner, Louis. "A Civil War Surgeon's Diary." *North Carolina Medical Journal* 27 (1966): 409–15.

Although a graduate of Jefferson Medical College, J. F. Shaffner enlisted as a private at the start of the Civil War. Later he was assistant surgeon of the 33rd and the 4th North Carolina, and later a brigade surgeon with the Army of Northern Virginia. He complained that his biggest problem was that the hatred men felt for him when he turned down their requests for medical furloughs. On 27 May 1862, he stayed behind with the wounded while other doctors rode off. He was taken by the Yankees, with his wounded, to Fortress Monroe. He was later released at City Point. January through March of 1864 were taken up by an argument with the regimental commanding officer and a subsequent court-martial. At the court-martial, he defended himself and was acquitted.

Sharpe, William D. "The Wounds of War, with Particular Reference to 1861–1865." *New York State Journal of Medicine* 85 (1985): 61–63.

This short article presents the effect of war upon body and mind. The first half describes the physical wounds made by minie balls, mainly with cases from Chisholm's *Manual.* The second half describes the psychological wounds of the Civil War and all wars that afflict the soldier, his family, and society.

Shryock, Richard H. *Medicine and Society in America, 1660–1860*. New York: New York University Press, 1960, 182 p.

Shryock was the leading medical historian when he wrote this short book. He argues that between the years 1790 and 1860, American medicine and medical care may actually have deteriorated. The medical profession changed from a few-well educated doctors, often with final training at Edinburgh or another major European university, to many poorly educated doctors who had obtained the M.D. degree after attending two series of lectures (actually one series given twice). Public health may have worsened during the period with an increasing mortality in large American cities. Medical therapy produced more symptoms than it relieved, leading to the appearance and success of groups of physicians wedded to special forms of medical practice. Although written thirty years ago, this book remains one of the best descriptions of the early years of American medicine.

Shryock, Richard H. "A Medical Perspective on the Civil War." *American Quarterly* 14 (1962): 161–73.

The dean of American medical historians was stimulated to survey Civil War medical history by the excessive (as he saw it) celebrations of the Civil War centennial. One must study the "incredible suffering which occurred on battlefields and in hospitals" in order to "guard against the assumption that all major outcomes in the American past must have been for the best." The American Civil War was among the bloodiest of wars because the large number of men engaged on both sides "sought out opponents with much determination." The minie balls of the era "did more damage than do modern, steel counterparts." The most appalling reason for the high mortality was slow evacuation; many soldiers bled to death or died of exposure. When their bodies were found days later, they were officially classified as killed in action. Shyrock thinks that the medical officers of the War were unnecessarily brutal. They may have been better doctors in their home communities, but now they were "practicing a form of state medicine," they "had neither the time nor inclination to cultivate solicitude or even bedside manners." Shyrock concludes that centennial celebrations should be balanced against the human misery of the War: "if medical aspects are omitted, the story is not only incomplete but is unrealistic." The author adds the opinion that if the conflict could have been postponed for two decades, the medical departments could have saved many more lives.

Shutes, Milton H. *Lincoln and the Doctors: A Medical Narrative of the Life of Abraham Lincoln.* New York: Pioneer Press, 1933, 152 p.

This book is a life of Lincoln with emphasis on the different doctors he knew. When living in New Salem, he knew quite well several doctors including Charles Chandler, Francis Regnier, and John Allen. In January of 1841, at the age of thirty-two, Lincoln wrote a long letter to the noted physician Daniel Drake, listing his symptoms and asking advice. Drake invited Lincoln to Cincinnati, but he could not go that far. Lincoln thought that his symptoms were due to hypochondriasis, and Shutes agrees. In Springfield, Lincoln knew Drs. John Todd and William Wallace, both kinsmen of Mary Todd. The book lists Lincoln's medication purchases from Diller's Drug Store. In 1857, Lincoln defended two doctors in his only malpractice action; not only did the doctors win, but the plaintiff had to pay all legal costs including Lincoln's fee. After his election to the presidency, Lincoln's doctor in Washington was Robert King Stone. The death of his son and Lincoln's illness after the Gettysburg Address are examined by Shutes.

The book concludes with the horrible night at Ford's Theater. The first person to minister to the wounded Lincoln was Dr. Charles A. Leale. Shutes had met Leale, who died 13 June 1932 at age ninety; in his later life, Leale refused to talk about that night, but he always saved his blood stained shirt. Other doctors who helped carry Lincoln to the Peterson house were Charles S. Taft and Alfred F. A. King. Surgeon General Joseph K. Barnes tried to extract the bullet. A large number of other doctors visited Lincoln in his last hours, including Charles H. Crane, Neal Hall, C. H. Lieberman, J. F. May, Beecher Todd, and E. W. Abbott.

Simkins, Francis Butler, and James Welch Patton. *The Women of the Confederacy.* Richmond: Garrett and Massie, 1936, 306 p.

This review of Southern women contains a chapter on hospital service.

Smith, Arthur M. "Getting Them Out Alive." *Naval Institute Proceedings* (February 1989): 41–46.

This article is a very interesting summary of the early or battle-field treatment of different forms of combat wounds, past and present. The author uses the term "meatball surgery" to describe hurried emergency treatment under combat conditions.

Smith, Dale C. "Quinine and Fever: The Development of the Effective Dosage." *Journal of the History of Medicine and Allied Sciences* 31 (1976): 343–67.

The value of quinine in malaria was muddied by the tendency to give too little. In 1847 Elisha Bartlett called quinine a "specific antiperiodic." By the time of the Civil War, medical science had determined that a dosage of about twenty grains given once per day would prevent malaria and three times per day would cure.

Smith, Dale C. "The Rise and Fall of Typhomalarial Fever." *Journal of the History of Medicine and Allied Sciences* 37 (1982): 182–200 and 287–321.

This essay is a very long discussion of how to classify patients who apparently have both malaria and typhoid fever. In 1898, most patients diagnosed as having typhomalarial fever were found at autopsy to have typhoid fever only.

Smith, Edward P. *Incidents of the United States Christian Commission.* Philadelphia: J. B. Lippincott, 1869, 512 p.

This book is a series of anecdotes and stories, each with an uplifting message. Many members of the Christian Commission provided service to the sick body as well as to the spirit, but the only hospital stories in this book relate to deathbed conversions.

Smith, George W. *Medicines for the Union Army: The United States Army Laboratories during the Civil War.* Madison, WI: American Institute for the History of Pharmacy, 1962, 119 p.

This is the standard history of medications in the United States Army. The Army Medical Department built its own pharmaceutical laboratories. The book contains much statistical material.

Smith, John David. "Kentucky Civil War Recruits: A Medical Profile." *Medical History* 24 (1980): 185–96.

This interesting article reviews the records of Kentucky doctors who performed induction physicals during the years 1863 to 1865. The author found the reports of eight of the nine doctors, one for each Congressional district, who were the medical representatives on the board of enrollment. All males from ages twenty to forty-five were subject to the draft. Those undergoing examinations were in one of four groups: (1) draftees, or individuals selected for military service; (2) enrollees, or individuals subject to the draft who asked for an examination to discover if they were physically fit for service; (3) recruits or volunteers, a very small group by this time in the War; and (4) substitutes, or men hired by draftees to take their places if found physically fit. In reviewing the records, the author found a wide range of diseases or conditions, diagnosed by these eight doctors, with very little agreement. The doctors noted that many of the people examined tried to feign illness. In every district, a greater percentage of black than of white draftees were found physically fit for military service, but the author does not try to determine if they were truly healthier, if they were less adept or less motivated to feign illness, or if the healthier whites were already in the army.

Snyder, Charles McCool. *Dr. Mary Walker, the Little Lady in Pants*. New York: Vantage Press, 1962, 166 p.

This biography of Dr. Walker includes two chapters on her Civil War service. She graduated from Syracuse Medical College in 1855, the only woman in her class. At the start of the Civil War, she applied to become a Union army physician, but was rejected despite interviews with Finley, R. C. Wood, Stanton, and eventually Lincoln. In October 1861, she served as a volunteer at the hospital located in the Patent Office building. The surgeon-in-charge, Dr. John N. Green made her his administrative assistant. Despite being a civilian, she wore the uniform of an assistant surgeon of the Union army. She went to Chattanooga late in 1863. Because of the unexpected death of the assistant surgeon of the 52nd Ohio, she was assigned to that position by General Thomas. Her name does not appear on that unit's official roll, but she did receive in a lump sum many months later pay for five months of service as acting assistant surgeon. Dr. Perrin, medical director of the Army of the Cumberland, ordered her to sit for a medical examining board; she failed the oral examination.

While treating civilians in the area of north Georgia near Chattanooga, she was captured by Confederate cavalrymen on 10 April 1864. She was taken to Castle Thunder Prison in Richmond where she refused to be vaccinated against smallpox. On 12 August 1864 she was exchanged. On 5 October 1864 she received a contract as an acting assistant surgeon and was assigned to the Women's Prison Hospital, Louisville. Her experience as a prisoner of the Confederacy helped her communicate with women prisoners of the Union. She was discharged on 15 June 1865 after service at the Orphans Home, Clarksville, Tennessee. She was awarded the Congressional Medal of Honor for meritorious service on 11 November 1865. In 1917, a review of such awards removed those unassociated with valor under fire. Dr. Snyder, still alive and still wearing trousers, refused to relinquish her medal. It was posthumously restored by Congress in 1977.

Stark, Richard Boies. "Surgeons and Surgical Care of the Confederate States Army." *Virginia Medical Monthly* 87 (1960): 230–41.

This essay is a very valuable survey of the problems and responses of the Medical Corps of the Confederate States Army. The author paints a generally successful response to the major Confederate medical problem, "the fierce handicap of physical paucity." Stark, a leading plastic surgeon, concludes that the efforts of the Medical Department helped "keep the drama alive far longer than the physical realities would permit." His suggestion that "victory eluded these valiant people by only a moment" is not developed.

Starr, Paul. *The Social Transformation of American Medicine.* New York: Basic Books, 1982, 514 p.

The author uses the Civil War as an analogy for the clash between medical sects, especially traditional medicine (allopathy) versus botanism, hydropathy, herbalism, and homeopathy. During the Civil War, he says, "the regulars dominated the military medical boards, and the homeopaths, in spite of congressional support, were unable to gain approval for military service." The author mentions, but does not emphasize, the role of the huge Union hospital system and its low mortality in the postwar growth of civilian hospitals and the movement for sanitation.

Steiner, Paul E. *Physician-Generals in the Civil War.* Springfield, IL: Charles C. Thomas, 1966, 194 p.

This interesting book surveys six Confederate and twenty-seven Union generals who had been physicians before the war. Only two men in the Medical Department were ranked as brigadier generals: Hammond and Barnes. According to Steiner, the Confederate Surgeon General was not officially an officer. The military units controlled by generals who were line officers but who had been doctors before the War were not healthier than other units.

Steiner, Paul E. *Disease in the Civil War: Natural Biological Warfare in 1861–1865.* Springfield, IL: Charles C. Thomas, 1968, 243 p.

This major work uses the undigested statistics of the *Medical and Surgical History* to examine the medical or epidemiological aspects of many separate campaigns.

Steiner, Paul E. *Medical-Military Portraits of Union and Confederate Generals.* Philadelphia: Whitmore Publishing Co., 1968, 342 p.

The author reviews the wounds and the illnesses of ten generals:

McClellan, Sherman, Hooker, McPherson, and Reynolds of the Union army and A. S. Johnston, Hood, Jackson, Ewell, and Forrest of the Confederate army. He brings a modern knowledge of medicine to the problem of the generals who died of wounds: Reynolds would not have been significantly hurt if he had been wearing a modern combat helmet at Gettysburg; Stonewall Jackson could have survived his wound and subsequent pneumonia with antibiotics; Albert Sydney Johnston could have been saved at Shiloh by good medical care then available. He also considers the physical diseases suffered by various generals: McClellan remained in his tent during a key period of the Peninsula campaign because of diarrhea. He also attempts psychiatric diagnoses with a bit less success. Many military histories describe the failures of various Civil War commanders; this book shows how physical and mental illnesses and wounds contributed to these failures of command. Anyone who wishes to understand the military history of the American Civil War must be intimately familiar with this work.

Steiner, Walter R. "A Physician's Experiences in the United States Sanitary Commission during the Civil War." *Charaka Club Proceedings* 10 (1941): 172–91.

The author's father held several positions with the United States Sanitary Commission, including inspector for the Army of the Potomac. He accompanied that army during May and June of 1864. On 8 June he recorded in his diary: "the men look perfectly exhausted, the results of this long campaign are beginning to show themselves in worn out nervous systems, in utter lack of energy and in emaciated faces."

Sterkx, H. E. *Partners in Rebellion: Alabama Women in the Civil War.* Rutherford, NJ: Farleigh Dickinson University Press, 1970, 238 p.

A survey of the activities of Alabama women includes one chapter on their medical activities. An example is Juliet Opie Hopkins, who traveled from Mobile to Richmond at the start of the war to organize hospitals for Alabama troops; at first, these institutions were financed by her husband from his personal fortune. When supervising the evacuation of Confederate wounded from the Battle of Seven Pines, she was herself wounded.

Sternberg, Martha L. *George Miller Sternberg: A Biography.* Chicago: American Medical Association, 1920, 331 p.

The author married George Sternberg in 1869. Her biography contains one chapter on his Civil War experiences. Sternberg graduated from the College of Physicians and Surgeons in New York in 1860. He appeared before the army examining board on 28 May 1861, received a high grade, and was appointed assistant surgeon in the regular (not volunteer) army. A long letter from Sternberg describes in detail his capture and escape at First Bull Run. In the Peninsula campaign, Sternberg was present at the battles of Gaines Mill and Malvern Hill; he developed typhoid fever and was evacuated from Harrison's Landing. After a period as executive officer of the general hospital at Portsmouth Grove, Rhode Island, he became assistant medical director in New Orleans. He spent the last year of the War in charge of the general hospital at Cleveland.

Steuart, R. D. "Surgeons of the Confederacy: William F. Steuart." *Confederate Veteran* 35 (1917): 218.

Dr. Steuart was a surgeon with the Army of Northern Virginia in a brigade commanded by his cousin, General G. H. Steuart.

Stevens, John K. "Hostages to Hunger: Nutritional Night Blindness in Confederate Armies." *Tennessee Historical Quarterly* 48 (1989): 131–43.

The author argues that by 1863 most Confederate soldiers were suffering from dietary deficiency of vitamin A. This deficiency is known today to produce night blindness. In night actions during the Civil War, this disorder could produce disaster. As an example, the author describes the night battle of Wauhatchie. Imagine a battle when one side can see but their opponents are blind.

Stewart, Miller J. *Moving the Wounded: Litters, Cacolets, and Ambulance Wagons, U.S., 1776–1876.* Fort Collins, CO: Old Army Press, 1979, 134 p.

This book is a well-illustrated survey of methods of removing the wounded from the battlefield. It covers the arguments concerning two-wheeled versus four-wheeled vehicles.

Stille, Alfred *Address before the Philadelphia County Medical Society Delivered February 11, 1963.* Philadelphia: Collins, 1863, 20 p.

At the time of this address, the author was the retiring president of the Philadelphia County Medical Society. He bemoaned his suspicion that New York was replacing Philadelphia as the major American center of scientific medicine. In the second half of the essay, the author describes his experience at an unnamed Philadelphia military hospital. He gives a very excellent description of the dominant malady, diarrhea. He thinks this progresses to dysentery and then, perhaps, to typhoid fever. The best treatment is a protected diet, basically of bread; patients who seem to have recovered develop diarrhea again when they attempt a general diet. He saw malaria responding well to cinchona. Scurvy caused leg swelling and ecchymoses. Lemon juice and fresh vegetables are helpful, but mild exercise and sunshine are also important. He thinks that medical authorities place "too much faith in drugs or, wanting that, in some indefinable sanitary influence of a hospital residence." The types of illnesses seen in a civilian hospital (Bright's disease, phthisis, and dropsy) are seldom seen in a military hospital. He also describes a neuralgia of the intercostal nerves in soldiers who carry a knapsack that is too heavy (this may be the first of many nerve compression disorders now discussed under the heading of occupational palsies).

Stille, Alfred. *Epidemic Meningitis or Cerebro-spinal Meningitis.* Philadelphia: Lindsay and Blakiston, 1867, 178 p.

The author does not specifically mention the Civil War but refers to well over forty papers on epidemic meningitis published by Americans during the years 1864 through 1866. This is the first monograph on this disorder.

Stille, Charles. *History of the United States Sanitary Commission.* New York: Hurd and Houghton, 1868, 553 p.

This is the final report of the United States Sanitary Commission. Allan Nevins (*The War for the Union,* 3: 317) calls it "one of the most interesting books produced by the war."

Stimson, Julia C., and Ethel C. S. Thompson. "Women Nurses with the Union Forces during the Civil War." *Military Surgeon* 62 (1928): 1–17, 208–30.

This interesting review of women nurses serving with the Union army contains long quotations from published works as well as from contemporary letters, orders, and circulars.

Stone, James L. "W. W. Keen: America's Pioneer Neurological Surgeon." *Neurosurgery* 17 (1985): 997–1010.

A review of Keen's life by a modern neurosurgeon contains considerable detail about his Civil War experiences at First and Second Manassas and at Philadelphia hospitals. His Civil War studies on nerve injuries with Mitchell "laid the foundations of modern neurological surgery."

Straight, William M. "The Pensacola Campaign Through a Nurse's Eye." *Florida Medical Association Journal* 56 (1969): 632–36.

The Union forces at Fort Pickens, located on an island in Pensacola Bay, exchanged long-range artillery fire with Confederate forces on the mainland through much of 1861 and 1862. The Union commander notified General Braxton Bragg that the mainland hospital was in the line of fire; the Confederate chose to interpret his suggestion that the hospital be moved as a "barbarous threat" to destroy it, "disgracefully violating the hospital flag." Nevertheless, the hospital patients were relocated. This article contains a letter from an unidentified nun, a member of the Sisters of Charity, who was a nurse at the Confederate hospital.

Street, James, Jr. "Under the Influence." *Civil War Times Illustrated* 27 (May 1988): 30–35.

The author describes many generals, North and South, whose minds were clouded by opium or by alcohol, sometimes taken on the prescription of a doctor. His major example is General John Bell Hood during the Tennessee campaign of 1864. The general was in terrible pain because of the severe nerve injury suffered at Gettysburg and because he had undergone amputation of the right leg after the Battle of Chickamauga. The author thinks that Hood was taking large amounts of morphine because of this pain and that his thought processes were affected, leading to the major errors at Spring Hill and at Franklin, Tennessee.

"Surgeons of the Confederacy: Henry J. Warmuth." *Confederate Veteran* 40 (1932): 383.

Warmuth graduated from Rush Medical College in Chicago in 1862 and immediately headed south. After serving briefly at Chimborazo Hospital, he was assigned to the Army of Tennessee. He was left with the wounded in Smyrna, Tennessee, after the retreat of Hood's army in December 1864. He was not released from prison until the following July.

T

Taylor, Frank H. *Philadelphia in the Civil War, 1861–1865*. Philadelphia: published by the city, 1913, 360 p.

A large section on Philadelphia General Hospitals gives their location and the names of the predominant physicians.

231

Thomas, Emory M. *The Confederate Nation, 1861–1865.* New York: Harper and Row, 1979, 384 p.

The best overall review of the Confederacy, this work makes no observations on Confederate medicine. The major thesis is that the Confederacy went through two stages: (1) an agricultural nation emphasizing localism and an economy based upon race slavery; and (2) a partly industrialized nation with a strong central government willing to give up slavery to survive. The real Confederate revolution was not secession, but this change, under war pressure, from the agricultural to the centralized state. Even if the Confederacy had won the Civil War, the old Southern way of life was gone.

Thompson, John D., and Grace Goldin. *The Hospital: A Social and Architectural History.* New Haven: Yale University Press, 1975, 349 p.

This work covers the hospital from ancient to modern times with emphasis upon its architecture. The pavilion hospitals built by both the North and the South during the American Civil War were derived from the British experience in the Crimea. This book is very valuable to anyone wanting the dimensions or the layout of a Civil War hospital.

Thompson, William Y. "The U.S. Sanitary Commission." *Civil War History* (1956): 41–63.

This essay describes the origin, development, and success of the United States Sanitary Commission. It includes many interesting details, such as: medical inspectors were paid $2 a day plus expenses; Olmstead personally directed the first hospital ship, the *Daniel Webster,* on the York River during the Peninsula campaign; the Commission spent $75,000 to support the Gettysburg hospitals, and a Field Relief Corps was established for the Army of the Potomac after the Gettysburg campaign. Of special note is a section on how the Sanitary Commission was able to transport supplies to Union soldiers in Confederate prisons.

Thompson, William Y. "Sanitary Fairs of the Civil War." *Civil War History* 4 (1958): 51–67.

This article describes in detail each fair, beginning with the Northwestern Sanitary Fair, held in Chicago from 27 October to 7 November 1863. Schools and courts were closed, and many people visited the exhibits at the fairgrounds. The fairs obtained money and material for distribution. Many clashes occurred; one, for example, was over whether or not to have raffles. Thompson concludes that the fairs were a financial success and helped to solidify support for the Union war effort.

Tiffany, Francis. *Life of Dorothea Lynde Dix*. Boston: Houghton Mifflin, 1896, 392 p.

This work is mainly about Dix's prewar career. In 1861, she was sixty years old and a world famous philanthropist and crusader for asylums for the insane and the blind. The chapter on the Civil War describes how Dix went to Secretary of War Simon Cameron in April 1861, after seeing the attack of the Baltimore mob upon the 6th Massachusetts, and was appointed Superintendant of Women Nurses. She selected nurses and sent them to various general hospitals where they were most needed. Many of her wartime letters are reproduced in full. She continued working throughout the War, never taking a single day off, but the author concludes that her most valuable service occurred before the United States Sanitary Commission was fully operational.

Tobey, James A. *The Medical Department of the Army: Its History, Activities and Organization*. Baltimore: Johns Hopkins University Press, 1927, 161 p.

This brief history of the United States Army Medical Department includes a summary of the Civil War experience. The book emphasizes laws and regulations, many taken verbatim from the earlier work by Ingersoll. Tobey makes a few interesting observations and evaluations. "The consensus of opinion among writers familiar with the work of this officer and the conditions of the times seems to be that Hammond was one of the great surgeon generals." Surgeon W. J. H. White, medical director of the 6th Corps, was killed in action at Antietam; he was the only regular army medical officer to lose his life in battle.

Todd, Gary L. "An Invalid Corps: Will the Wounded Serve?" *Civil War Times Illustrated* 24 (December 1985): 10–19.

This article describes the Invalid Corps of the Union army. Individuals about to receive a medical discharge could be transferred to this corps, where they could perform limited duty such as guarding prison camps. Each of the eventual sixteen regiments of the corps consisted of six companies of soldiers who could perform most duties not requiring strenuous labor (the first battalion) and four companies of soldiers with more severe disabilities such as loss of an arm (the second battalion). The Corps was formed on 28 April 1863 and merged into the Veteran Reserve Corps on 18 March 1864. The Veteran Reserve Corps included soldiers who were not disabled but who were eligible for discharge from their original regiments because of expiration of term of service. On 21 March 1865, the Veteran Reserve Corps was reorganized; all twenty-four of its regiments consisted of soldiers who were fit enough to be in the first battalion. The more seriously disabled soldiers of the second battalion were all transferred to the control of the surgeon general of the Army and served as hospital attendants.

Tomes, Nancy. "The Private Side of Public Health: Sanitary Science, Domestic Hygiene, and the Germ Theory, 1870–1900." *Bulletin of the History of Medicine* 64 (1990): 509–39.

The author thinks that the major decrease in infectious disease mortality that began in the United States in the decade of the 1870s resulted from the popularization of sanitary science. After a generation of middle-class voters had been educated in proper hygienic practices, "public health authorities were able more effectively to impose those same practices on the poor, under the aegis of state medicine." The author discusses the educational techniques of public health authorities in detail, but never mentions the experience of the general population with hygiene during the Civil War.

Trudeau, Noah Andre. *Bloody Roads South: The Wilderness to Cold Harbor, May–June 1864*. Boston: Little Brown, 1989, 354 p.

This book summarizes the Union efforts in Virginia in the summer of 1864. A chapter surveys the evacuation of the wounded after the Battle of the Wilderness, fought 5 through 7 May. The first stop was Rappahannock Station, then by rail or wagons to Fredericksburg, and finally by rail to ship to Washington. The system functioned well, with Washington receiving over 14,000 wounded by 18 May.

U

Underwood, John Levi. *The Women of the Confederacy*. New York: Neale Publishing, 1906, 313 p.

This book contains snippets gathered from many sources. Several of the anecdotes concern female nurses such as Phoebe Pember, Mrs. Pryor, and Sally Tompkins.

W

Wade, David R. "Starting Largely with the Civil War, French Captain Minie's Invention Revolutionized Warfare." *America's Civil War* 1 (July 1988): 8.

This brief essay summarizes the effects of the minie ball and how it changed warfare.

Wangensteen, Owen H., Jacqueline Smith, and Sarah D. Wangensteen. "Some Highlights in the History of Amputation Reflecting Lessons in Wound Healing." *Bulletin of the History of Medicine* 41 (1967): 97–131.

This scholarly and massive review of amputation includes a large section on the Civil War. During the War, most surgeons left the stump open; it closed by the development of granulation tissue over a period of many months. A few surgeons attempted to suture the stump closed after amputation; if the sutures held, healing was much faster, but most often suppuration occurred, breaking open the wound. The authors state that modern studies have shown that this attempt to suture the stump (called primary closure) is successful only if done within six to eight hours of the initial injury. The guillotine or open method was the only type of amputation performed in the World Wars.

Wangensteen, Owen H., and Sarah D. Wangensteen. *The Rise of Surgery: From Empiric Craft to Scientific Discipline*. Minneapolis: University of Minnesota Press, 1978, 785 p.

This massive tome covers the entire history of surgery. It is not strictly chronological, but is arranged by topic, such as types of operation or subspecializations of surgery. In the chapter on disinfectants, the authors state that many Civil War doctors used various materials to prevent gangrene or erysipelas from traveling from one wound to another. These include Middleton Goldsmith (bromine), George P. Hachenberg (turpentine), and Julian Chisolm and William Detmold (nitric acid). The chapter on war surgery discusses extensively the experiences of the American Civil War.

Waring, Joseph I. *A History of Medicine in South Carolina, 1825–1900*. Columbia: South Carolina Medical Association, 1967, 366 p.

This major work includes a chapter on the Civil War, covering both Confederate and Union activities. An appendix summarizes the lives of many leading South Carolina physicians, including J. J. Chisolm, David C. DeLeon, and Samuel P. Moore.

Warner, John Harley. "A Southern Medical Reform: The Meaning of the Antebellum Argument for Southern Medical Education." *Bulletin of the History of Medicine* 57 (1983): 364–81.

The author argues that, in the 1850s, Southern physicians began a reform movement to improve medical education in their region and to convince Southern youth to study at Southern medical institutions. They argued that Southern medical problems were different from the type of medical problems seen in the northern United States and Europe. Only local study over many generations would bring true improvement in Southern health.

White's Conspectus of American Biography: A Tabulated Record of American History and Biography, 2d edition. New York: James T. White and Co., 1937, 455 p.

This volume can be used as an index to the *National Cyclopedia of American Biography.* Lists of prominent American physicians and military surgeons include many individuals with important Civil War service.

Wickham, Julia P. "Francis Peyre Porcher: Physician, Botanist, Author." *Confederate Veteran* 33 (1925): 456–59.

The author describes the Civil War career of her father, who wrote a botanical manual for the Confederacy, listing the flora of the Southern nation that might be of medical use.

Wiley, Bell Irvin. *The Life of Billy Yank: The Common Soldier of the Union,* and his *The Life of Johnny Reb: The Common Soldier of the Confederacy.* Indianapolis, IN: Bobbs-Merrill, 1951, 454 p., and 1943, 444 p.

These classic works upon the everyday life of the common soldiers each contain a chapter upon sickness and medical care.

Wilkinson, Warren. *Mother, May You Never See the Sight I Have Seen: The 57th Massachusetts Veteran Volunteers in the Army of the Potomac, 1864–1865.* New York: Harper and Row, 1990, 665 p.

This book on the 57th Massachusetts during the Virginia campaign of 1864–65 contains a chapter on the handling of the wounded after the Battle of the Wilderness. Many specific cases are described with eyewitness accounts of their evacuation and treatment in Fredericksburg. A section on members of the regiment who became prisoners at Andersonville relies on the diary of Austin K. Gould, who was a doctor, but not a medical officer.

Wise, E. Robert "Life and Times of Samuel Preston Moore, Surgeon General of the Confederate States of America." *Southern Medical Journal* 22 (1930): 916–22.

This article is written with authority and based upon published material and personal communications. Born in Charleston in 1813, Moore graduated from the medical school there in 1824. His twenty-six years in the United States Army included service in the Mexican War and throughout the west. After resignation on 25 February 1861, he practiced medicine in Little Rock. Jefferson Davis, however, appointed him Surgeon General on 7 November 1861. After the War he never practiced medicine again, but was involved with the Virginia State Fair and the Richmond School Board, during which time he introduced compulsory vision testing for school children. He died 31 May 1889. He organized the Medical Department against great difficulties. He obtained medical books from retired practitioners or their widows and sent them to physicians in the field. He directed the publication of the important *Manual* of 1863 and published the Confederate medical journal. "A very remarkable achievement," Wise concludes.

Wise, Stephen R. *Lifeline of the Confederacy: Blockade Running during the Civil War.* Columbia: University of South Carolina Press, 1988, 403 p.

This is the major work on the effect of the naval blockade upon the Confederacy. The appendices describe ship arrivals and ship losses with encyclopedic throroughness. The author concludes that the blockade did not play a major role in the defeat of the Confederacy because some items—even luxury items such as gowns from Paris—continued to slip into Southern ports. The book makes no statement on the shortage of quinine.

Wodehouse, Lawrence. "John McArthur Jr (1823–1890)." *Journal of the Society of Architectural Historians* 28 (1969): 271–83.

John McArthur, Jr. was a well-known architect of public buildings at the outbreak of the War. He designed twenty-four temporary United States Army hospitals, including the huge Mower Hospital at Chestnut Hill, Philadelphia.

Z

Zeidenfelt, Alex. "The Embattled Surgeon-General, William A. Hammond." *Civil War Times Illustrated* 17 (October 1978): 24–32.

This article reviews Hammond's struggle with the Secretary of War, ending with his court-martial.

Zellem, Ronald T. "Wounded by Bayonet, Ball, and Bacteria: Medicine and Neurosurgery in the American Civil War." *Neurosurgery* 17 (1985): 850–60.

This article is a detailed summary of the treatment of combat injuries during the Civil War with special emphasis on head injuries.

Zone, Robert M. "Venereal Diseases: A Historical Perspective." *Journal of the Tennessee Medical Association* 81 (1988): 451–53.

Syphilis and gonorrhea were significant problems among the Union troops occupying Nashville and Memphis. Military authorities in Nashville loaded all the prostitutes of the city upon a steamer bound for Louisville, but they were all back within a month. The Union military government licensed all prostitutes who passed a medical examination and paid 50 cents per week as a special tax to support a hospital where prostitutes with signs of venereal disease could be kept until healthy. Each woman received a certificate of health to show to her customers. The rate of venereal disease fell markedly until November of 1863, when Sherman's troops marched overland from Memphis to the relief of Chattanooga. Each regiment spent only a day or two in Nashville while en route, but this was long enough to reinfect the city's prostitutes. After this, however, venereal disease was soon brought again under control in Nashville; Memphis introduced a similar system. Civilian authorities in both cities did not like to be associated with a system that licensed prostitutes and the end of military law terminated this experiment in venereal disease control.

INDEX

241

243

248

250

251